The
Connected
THERAPIST

RELATING THROUGH THE SENSES

MARTI SMITH, OTR/L

Published by Marti Smith Seminars, Inc.

Print ISBN: 978-1-7372052-0-3

http://www.creativetherapies.com

I'm a better therapist because I've known Marti Smith. When I sent my clients and their families to work with Marti, they were loved and cared for in the same way she loves and cares for her reader in The Connected Therapist. Marti is gifted in helping parents and caregivers see their child through a new lens -the body-awakening curiosity in even the most frustrated adult. *The Connected Therapist* draws the reader in with story and then packs their toolbox with simple, every day interventions. I want every parent I know to read this book.

Robyn Gobbel
LMSW-Clinical

Table of Contents

Introduction
Foreword

INTRODUCTION

I've heard the phrase, "You should write a book" countless times. My life is full of interesting characters, compelling settings, crazy adventures, and plenty of conflicts in need of resolution. But, in the same way that some faces are meant for radio, my words are meant for the stage. A stage doesn't need spell check or commas. And a book doesn't have the benefit of tone of voice or an appropriate pause before the punchline.

To be a good writer, it helps to be a good reader. But I prefer to live my own stories rather than reading about someone else's. I'd rather be camping, skiing, baking cookies or taking photos than sitting at my keyboard deciding between "there" and "their." I'm a math savant who took remedial English classes. Write a book? Me?

My friend Sarah Mercado once told me, "You may be singing the same song as others, but you will have your own version, and the more people who are singing, the more people get to hear the music."

So...I wrote a book. My personal and professional experience combined with my knowledge of the brain give me insight into people who have experienced adversity, especially children. As an occupational therapist, I've spent decades working with children and families. I've found it extremely gratifying to hear from countless parents and teachers that I've helped them with a child in their care.

At the time of this writing, Oprah Winfrey and Dr. Bruce Perry have just published a new book titled *What Happened to You?: Conversations on Trauma, Resilience, and Healing.* If they are musicians playing a sold-out concert, then I'm a street performer singing a Dr. Perry song under a bridge in Austin. But I've decided to sing it all the same.

Children have inherent worth regardless of how society might try to quantify their development. This isn't a book about helping parents raise perfect kids. It's a book about loving imperfect people, ourselves included. It's about being compassionate, having empathy, and doing the best we can while striving to learn more, because when we *know* better, we *do* better.

I'm grateful for those who have joined my band along the way. Holly Timberline is an OT from my trauma-informed OT group who helped me edit for both content and grammar. I could not have completed this book without her. Dr. Cross, Dr. Perry, and Michael Remole encouraged me to share my perspective. Dr. Kelly Mahler and Marc Dingman, PhD answered my cold call for help with the interoceptive and proprioceptive content.

Plenty of people love the symphony. But plenty also love a laid-back street performer like me. I hope you're one of them, and I hope my song stays in your head and that you think of it when you need it most.

FOREWORD

A little over two years ago I had a heart attack, which led to open heart surgery and a triple bypass. What I didn't know at the time, was that my surgeon was one of the best in North Texas, and I was fortunate to have him. The more I learned about this man, from talking to him (he is not only smart, but warm and caring), from others who know him and his work, and from what I have read about him in various magazines, I have come to believe that he is a marvelous instrument for doing good. Now, I understand that we don't usually think of people as "instruments" — after all, aren't the instruments in this case his scalpel and other tools he has at his disposal while doing surgery? I would call those the tools of his trade, but he is the true instrument. He is the one who brings the whole enterprise together into the magic of surgery done well — all of the tools, machines, and team of medical professionals that supports him. He is an instrument of excellence, an instrument for doing something profoundly good and complex.

For many of the same reasons I would say that Marti Smith is an instrument, an instrument whose excellence almost seems to be divinely inspired. I chose to open this foreword with the example of a medical professional, in part because I know Marti comes from a medical family, and this example would be meaningful to her. But I also chose the example because I think it is easier for us to appreciate the skill and expertise of the surgeon (think of all the exposure we get from TV shows like *ER* and *Grey's Anatomy*), whereas we may not know so much about the skill and expertise of the occupational therapist. That said, I know firsthand that the numerous families that Marti has served are fully aware of Marti's healing magic and believe her to be divinely sent.

As an instrument, in the sense I am using the word here, my heart surgeon fused together knowledge from many sources into a singular practice. As an instrument, Marti has done the same thing. Three sources of knowledge and expertise stand out. The first is Marti's own personal experience, which is derived from her journey as a child, a woman, a parent, a wife, a friend, and a professional. Her journey has not been easy — it has been a warrior's journey — but like most journeys, it has been one full of lessons for someone willing to learn. One of the things I love about this book is that Marti weaves together her personal and professional journeys, and it's this weaving that has helped make Marti the instrument she has become. It also reveals a profound truth about what makes a fine instrument: You can't separate the personal from the professional.

A second source of knowledge and experience for Marti has been her close association with Dr. Bruce Perry and the ChildTrauma Academy. Dr. Perry is the world's foremost child traumatologist, and no one understands the impact of relational trauma on children better than he. Dr. Perry's wisdom has been distilled into his Neurosequential Model of Therapeutics™ (NMT), which has become one of the cornerstones of trauma-informed assessment and practice in the world today. Marti is herself a highly valued trainer in the model, and one of the things that makes her special is her ability to seamlessly integrate the NMT framework into her consulting and training practice. The NMT model, when it is properly applied and understood, provides extraordinary insight into the root causes of the many challenging behaviors that we too often find in traumatized children and youth. Using a phrase from our own work at the KPICD, the NMT model provides a platform for professionals to "See the need," so that they can "Meet the need."

A third source of knowledge and experience for Marti has been her close association with Dr. Karyn Purvis, myself, and the staff at the KPICD here at Texas Christian University. Marti has trained as a Practitioner in the KPICD's trauma-informed model, Trust-Based Relational Intervention (TBRI). Whereas Bruce Perry's NMT model provides tools for "seeing what and where the need is," TBRI provides tools for "meeting the need." Marti has proven to be highly adept — an exquisite instrument — at blending the knowledge and skills of NMT with those of TBRI, and then blending both therapeutic models with her knowledge and expertise as an occupational therapist. All of this combined with her passion and personal insight makes for a potent blend. And from this comes her book, *The Connected Therapist*, which is a gift. This book is a close cousin of *The Connected Child*, similar in the value it has for parents and professionals. But it is also different. Whereas there is no shortage of insight in *The Connected Child*, Marti's book reflects a more mature understanding of relational trauma, its impact, and how to heal its wounds and scars.

The field has come far since *The Connected Child* was written, and Marti's book reflects this more mature understanding, while at the same time preserving the accessibility of the earlier book.

Marti Smith, herself an exquisite instrument for healing, has produced a book worthy of her practice. *The Connected Therapist* is a tool that the rest of can use to improve our own practices, whether we are practicing as parents or as professionals, or both.

David R. Cross, Ph.D
Rees-Jones Director of the Karyn Purvis
Institute of Child Development and
Professor, Department of Psychology,
Texas Christian University

Becoming Connected

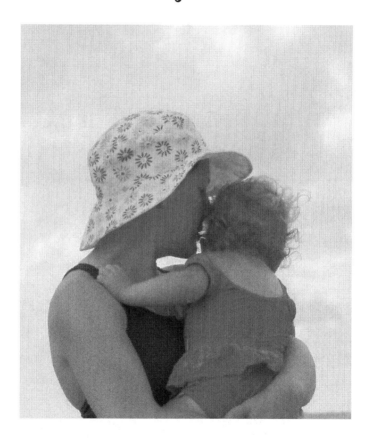

CHAPTER 1

FROM DISSOCIATION TO CONNECTION

In September 2007 I was on vacation at a beach with my husband and two-year-old daughter. I had just completed a Bible study based on Beth Moore's book, *Breaking Free*. Beth writes in that book about breaking the chains of generational sin and her words burned my soul as much as the hot Texas sun beating down on my skin. Beth's idea that my ancestors' decisions affected me, and my parenting, was eye opening. I was determined not to walk the same path as those who walked before me. I saw women in my life being treated unkindly at times and witnessed the effects of their various coping mechanisms. To avoid their hurt feelings, they threw themselves into proving their value through physical appearance, work accomplishments, avoiding close relationships, and retreating into themselves. I saw myself using those same coping mechanisms while raising my own child. As I started researching epigenetics and trauma for my work, I began to understand those coping mechanisms as symptoms of each generation coping with their own histories of trauma, dissociation, and disconnected

1

relationships.

This is a story about my journey from dissociation to connection, and how the things I learned along the way now help me light the path for others. How I am attempting to "break the generational chains" of my own heritage. How this breaking of the chains has empowered me in my personal, professional, and therapeutic relationships. How my own study of epigenetics, family beliefs, cultural patterns, and attachment styles has greatly changed my own parenting, and ultimately how I work as an occupational therapist who specializes in somatosensory activity recommendations for children who have experienced adversity.

In my studies, I was introduced to the term "dissociation" by a trauma expert, Dr. Bruce D. Perry, MD, PhD. Dr. Perry utilizes a model called the Arousal Continuum which describes how the body moves between the states of calm to terror. In this model, he describes dissociation as a way to protect the body from feeling intense emotional hurt or physical pain. Dissociation can be protective against physical injury. If our muscles have less movement and blood flow, we will bleed out slower if a tiger bites off our limb. Women and small children especially tend to dissociate as a survival skill. Biologically, they are less able to fight back, so they withdraw within themselves.

But dissociation isn't just physical. Research indicates that we dissociate cognitively throughout our day. During a conversation or teaching lesson (even while reading this book), we may dissociate every ten to twenty seconds. Our brain takes quick input breaks as we decide which information goes to memory and which information is no longer needed to move forward. If we had to process every piece of information we encountered, our brains would be overloaded and inefficient.

We need dissociation to reach a state of rest and recovery. Some people have to read a book before bed to turn off their brain. Some people pray or meditate. These mental breaks keep us alive. They keep us sane. But when we retreat into them too often, it becomes hard to connect with those around us.

As I looked at my own familial coping strategies, I realized that many of my relatives were dissociating for protection — at the expense of connection. When my mother would go for nine-mile prayer walks each day, she was able to get a break from her personal stress. But that made being a connected caregiver difficult. I saw divorce, infidelity, drug use, abandonment, excessive exercise, and workaholism. I also saw these dissociative patterns in myself. When we can't connect with people, we will connect with other things. As my journey continued, I began to understand how connection through human relationships is key to rehabilitating these dissociative patterns.

One of the things that impacted my own journey was completing training in Trust-Based Relational Intervention (TBRI) to become a TBRI Practitioner. TBRI is an attachment-based intervention focused on empowering, connecting, and correcting. Dr. Karyn Purvis co-created this intervention with Dr. David Cross and taught that "we cannot bring a child to a place of healing that we have not been ourselves." Prior to that training, I didn't understand that I would have to do my own healing before I could help others. With master dissociative skills, I easily separated my own feelings and background from my work with others. I had yet to learn that my "dismissive-avoidant" attachment style hindered my attachment not only to my own child, but also to the families with whom I worked.

Granted, being dismissive avoidant is a great skill when you are interested in human dissection and gross anatomy. So I'm glad I learned to attach better after I learned all that stuff in school. I'm grateful for the timing of that personal growth. I'm also encouraged by it. In our youth, the stupid blunders give us good stories that carry us through our more cautious and dull older years. We don't have to know everything from the start. Indeed, how boring would life be without those blunders? I hope to have really entertaining stories of all the mistakes I've made that led to learning and improvements when I'm older.

Although I was determined to break the dissociative cycle within my family, I was failing miserably. I had spent my twenties happily dissociating into my very rewarding career as an occupational therapist specializing in autism. I had no childhood dreams of becoming a mother and had been told I would never have children. Therefore, I was shocked to find out I was pregnant at age thirty. At the very appointment where my oncologist told me my new "tumor has a heartbeat," I was also told that, given my health issues, I probably wouldn't carry that baby to term. I maintained a healthy lifestyle, but I wasn't exactly preparing for parenthood. No nursery, no dreams or excitement over something I would likely miscarry. With all the trauma I was experiencing through my pregnancy,

I remained disconnected and dissociated from the reality that I was about to be a mother. I spent thirty-four weeks of pregnancy preparing for a loss that never happened. Then, after an emergency C-section, I had a baby. I was a child specialist, and I felt completely unprepared to parent. **I was looking for a way to break the dissociative cycle without any frame of reference or support on how to actually do it.**

When we returned from that September beach trip, my husband met a man who would drastically change the course of our parenting. But it would be two years before my own introduction to him. It took two years because at that time, I was newly pregnant. Again. I was full of hormones and exhausted trying to meet the needs of a very fussy little one while also dealing with morning sickness. So, when Dr. Bruce Perry connected with my husband, a gifted software developer, upon our return from vacation, I paid very little attention. Bruce wanted him to write some new metric that was similar to a brain map but based on behaviors instead of electrical impulses. My husband kept asking me to be involved in this work and I kept pushing back. I couldn't focus on his new little "side job." I was in the world of autism, not trauma. I was also feeling hopeful, overwhelmed, and excited to be newly pregnant. But just a few months later, **I was grieving the loss of that baby. I had connected with that new life inside my belly while struggling to connect with the child in my arms**. Working in childhood trauma seemed depressing and triggering to me. My childhood was full of trauma and my own motherhood experience wasn't exactly delightful.

I wasn't persuaded to participate in this project until

Bruce called my husband one night when a friend of mine was over. Julie Kouri is an inspiring adoptive family advocate, and she was impressed that my husband was casually chatting with the leading expert in childhood trauma research. She urged me to collaborate with Dr. Perry, the same way that my husband, Rob, had been doing for two years:

"It's about the brain," Rob would say. "You love that stuff!"

"Dr. Perry could use more sensory strategies," Julie would say. "You love that stuff!"

Saying yes (finally!) to my husband's introduction significantly changed the course of my career trajectory. Since joining the Neurosequential Model of Therapeutics (NMT) community and becoming a fellow at ChildTrauma Academy in 2010, my focus has shifted to helping families with children who have experienced adversity. As my career focus changed to trauma, I began to find the tools to heal my own family.

Dr. Perry was interested in my work with autism and in the trainings and tactics I'd developed to help calm sensory systems. I had an in-depth understanding of human anatomy, neurology, and what are known as the hidden senses. I also had a great gift of making things easy to understand while finding creative and inexpensive activities to meet my clients' goals. He was keen to bring me onto his team and mentioned international travel. Now we were talking! Travel is a favorite hobby for master dissociators. A chance to physically and geographically remove myself from my life's problems? Sign me UP! I was ready to travel.

As it turned out, though, I wasn't ready for the ways that Dr. Perry's training videos rocked my world. My view of childhood trauma was crack houses, abuse, neglect, and violence. I had personal experience with some of that. But to me, that wasn't real trauma. It was just how we lived. I knew it wasn't normal, but I didn't consider it trauma. There are still times when my husband will tell me, "You know, that's not normal" when I describe events of my childhood. For instance, my siblings and I were locked in a room for long periods of time. We were noisy, and the adults needed quiet, so shutting us in a room and locking the door seemed perfectly reasonable to us. We always went in willingly. Sometimes we would sneak in food, but we never questioned the lock-ups. I don't think the adults even considered it abuse. They just wanted to make sure we were safe while they were unavailable. Now, as an adult, I can understand how children can endure some kinds of neglect or abuse and not think to tell anyone. I have firsthand experience of how "normal" is truly relative. It all depends on who you are related to and how they raised you.

I was sure there was no trauma in my adult life. I had years of counseling and was determined to work towards healthier relationships. An ex-boyfriend once told me, "You know what I like about you, Marti? You've got a lot of baggage. But you've managed to pack it neatly into a carry-on." **My husband will now further express that while I did have nice carry-on luggage, I failed to mention to him the many delivery boxes that I had shipped ahead that**

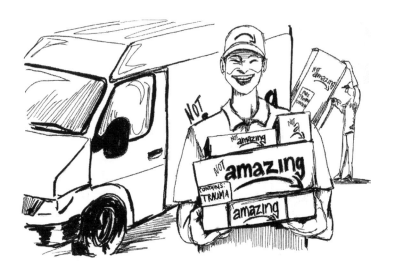

would show up later in our marriage.

I hadn't even considered how my own four-year-old daughter could be labeled as having a trauma background. How could her life in an upper-middle-class white family who met her needs be considered traumatic? I hadn't considered that her inability to soothe and colicky behavior wasn't just because she was a "sensory kid." I was a sensory kid! I figured it was all part of the genetic lottery. I didn't understand how "sensory issues" could be related to birth trauma or attachment styles. The training videos showed me that my own emotional and health issues while pregnant, and the emergency circumstances of her birth, indeed qualified her as a "trauma kid."

As the puzzle pieces finally created a coherent picture, my maternal guilt also came into sharp focus, and I was a wreck. I now understood why some of my purely sensory strategies were not working—not only for my own daughter, but also for many of my clients with early adverse experiences. I knew that in breaking the chains of my ancestors, I was being called to break the chains for others who, like me, didn't even know they were bound.

I have a few goals for this book. I hope you will find it entertaining. I love a good story and I've lived a life full of good stories to tell. But more than just entertaining you, I hope it inspires you. In the chapters that follow, I hope you can see a little of yourself or the children you love in these stories. I hope I can offer you new insights into the "why" behind puzzling behaviors. I hope you discover new strategies to try. I hope this book gives you empathy and compassion for yourself and others and reminds you that we are all simply doing the best we can with what we know. I hope if my relatives ever read this, they know that I believe with all my heart they were doing the best they could with the circumstances they were in.

In a moment of me being judgmental, my stepmom heard me criticize a family member for not being sober enough to get out of the car for the burial of their child. I said, "I just can't imagine how they couldn't even say goodbye." My stepmom quietly replied, "By the grace of God, you can't." Those wise and convicting words have stuck with me. In my work, I hear many stories of horror that I can't possibly understand. But now I try to remember to be grateful for that lack of understanding, and to remind myself that we are all doing the best we can with what we have. My passion now is to help caregivers develop the skills to make better choices.

Over the years, I've seen the power of forgiveness, love,

healing, and reconciliation. I love Maya Angelou's quote, "You do the best you can until you know better. Then you do better.

1 hope each day, as I learn new things, I do better.

1 hope I help others better and treat others better.

1 hope maybe this book brings new friends together. Friends who will support each other like my friends have done over the decades.

1 hope this book connects people to themselves and to others.

1 hope it gives you a better understanding of the development of the sensory system and the implications of adverse experiences.

1 hope it helps you understand your own history and how that affects your parenting and care for others.

1 hope it gives you some practical strategies to help calm or alert the children you work with and love.

CHAPTER 2

MOVING FROM BEHAVIOR MANAGEMENT TO RELATIONAL UNDERSTANDING

As I immersed myself in understanding Dr. Perry's Neurosequential Model of Therapeutics, I found myself nodding along knowingly at many of the diagrams, case studies, and anatomical explanations he included. I've always loved anatomy. My father is a physician and some of my favorite memories were of hanging out with him in the ER. In the 1980s, things weren't as regulated and it was completely normal for my siblings and me to be dropped off in the doctor's lounge to entertain ourselves while Dad worked in a small rural hospital.

This is another example of the relativity of "normal." My childhood included hanging out in a hospital, jumping into a pool from a rooftop, riding motorcycles on a track in our front yard, attempting to add a basement using a hand shovel, and being told to keep the Cessna 150 airplane "where you can see I-70" at age ten, while dad napped on the way home.

Learning that "normal" is subjective has transformed how I view some of the children I work with. I've had many children from neglectful backgrounds who smear their feces. I tended to view this behavior from a tactile or attention-seeking perspective. While this is a useful perspective, learning to view normal as a repetitive neural activity opened my eyes. I have a vivid third-grade memory of wearing a sweatshirt that had not been washed since a visit with my father. One of the popular girls leaned over and told me I smelled. I took a big whiff and was immediately transported to my father's house. What repulsed my classmate just smelled like home to me.

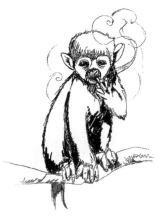

The funny thing about this story is I smelled like monkey pee and cigarettes. Because, for me, it was normal to live with monkeys and a parent who smoked. Monkeys who were supposed to stay in their cages but were excellent escape artists. Monkeys who would pee on you when you put them back in their cages. Yup, monkey piss and cigarettes — that was *my* normal.

My old love of anatomy gradually fused with a new understanding of how our neural pathways are formed and how the olfactory sense is a strong emotional connector. That's when I started to see how maybe the fecal smearers were actually comforted by the smell of their feces. Maybe they were left in their dirty diapers for long periods of time. Maybe the finger painting that they were able to entertain themselves with brought them some sort of comfort. Maybe this "smearing" simply brought them home, like my sweatshirt did for me. Re-framing how memories are made and how we perceive "normal" opened my therapeutic eyes to more possibilities of why children might engage in different types of sensory behaviors.

The sensory aspects of food and eating also form deep ties to childhood. As a child, it seemed to me like my dad was always working. If I wanted to see him, I went to the hospital. We even had a standing family tradition of eating Sunday brunch at the cafeteria. The menu never changed: chicken, mashed potatoes, green beans, and a roll. If you were extra lucky, you got a fountain soda and Jell-O, too. Some of my favorite family conversations happened in that hospital cafeteria. It was a predictable routine. Even in college, I visited my dad in that cafeteria. Sometimes that was the only way to really get his attention and have a conversation with him.

To this day, hospital food is my comfort food. That is my childhood normal. If I'm homesick, give me string beans and chicken. Please don't put ANY seasoning on it.

Can you see how your own ties to certain foods evolved, and how food and comfort and childhood memories become so intertwined? (There will be more on this later in the book.) After lunch, dad would have to do rounds. As we got older, he often would let us shadow him. I imagine that is why so many of his children ended up in medicine. It is a part of our heritage. It is our normal.

Dad was my personal Gregory House from the television show, *House*. His brilliance was tangible. He could diagnose things no one else saw. And he had a unique bedside manner.

"Doc, it hurts when I do this."

"Then don't do it."

This was a common banter out in the community when people approached him with their questions. Dad didn't always say a lot of words. But you could tell he was always thinking.

I loved being able to watch him sew someone up or deliver a baby via C-section. My childhood gave me such a unique window into human anatomy and biology. Even now, my software developer husband laughs at how often our family gatherings become a "who saw what weird diagnosis" event. My childhood experience is what led me to beg my OT school to enroll me in gross anatomy with the physical therapists. I'd studied the books and seen some live surgeries. But I wanted to get my hands on the anatomical structures and feel them. Understand them. Deeply study them. That's my normal.

I even wanted to dissect my children's deceased pet mouse to discover if there was a tumor on the spinal cord that caused his paralysis. Thankfully, my husband realized that pet mouse dissection wasn't everyone's normal. I credit him for shielding our children from the trauma of finding their mother mid-autopsy of their beloved Ben.

When I first started working with Dr. Perry, I was focused on my job as the OT. I was asked to provide sensory strategies for others learning his neurosequential model. I enjoyed Dr. Perry's teachings, but I didn't initially see them as transferable to the field of occupational therapy. The focus in my early trainings was on development, anatomy, and attachment theory. There was a lot of discussion about what behaviors or functions fit anatomically within a brain heuristic. These were things I had studied and mastered in neuroanatomy and OT school. It wasn't until several years later that I realized I had as much to learn about trauma as I had to teach about sensory processing. Occupational therapy is a career that, like nursing or teaching, can specialize in different settings. One of my best friends has the same degree as me but specializes in the hand. Not all OTs graduate with a deep understanding of how the sensory system develops. Even fewer OTs graduate with an understanding of how trauma impacts these developing systems. I am writing this book in hopes of inviting conversations and sharing knowledge between caregivers, counselors, teachers, and therapists to help build compassion and inspire trauma-informed collaborations. To maximize the benefits of occupational therapy for children who have experienced adversity, caregivers need to understand how the sensory system functions. Therapists need to understand how trauma impacts the sensory system and relationships within the context of family and community.

In the 2010s, thirty to sixty minutes of therapy in a gym,

separate from caregivers, was standard. Insurance treated it as reimbursable. Clients even made gains, which allowed me to update my goals in my progress reports. But I was missing the fact that every action, every thought, every FUNCTIONAL movement was a neural firing. It was something I "knew." But I didn't "KNOW" it. It didn't resonate deeply. Only when this piece clicked into place did I realize that I needed to embrace caregivers as treatment team members. How much better could my outcomes be if the caregivers were able to carry over my treatment daily? What if those functional neural firings could happen with more repetition than just the thirty minutes a week inside my treatment gym? What if they could happen within the context of a consistent and connected relationship?

It was about this time, in 2013, that my friend Julie Kouri (the same friend who encouraged me to connect with Dr. Perry) introduced me to Dr. Karyn Purvis. Dr. Purvis seemed intrigued that I was connected with Dr. Perry and had a decent grasp on the sensory system. I was also starting to understand how trauma fit in the puzzle of complex clinical diagnostics. Dr. Purvis agreed to allow me to sit in on the newly forming Travis County Collaborative for Trust-Based Relational Intervention. It was a room full of judges, teachers, social workers, bus drivers, juvenile justice workers, counselors, and even equine professionals. I was the only OT and I met some amazing friends and colleagues that day. It was here that I first learned how many of us in the caregiving professions have our own trauma histories.

I had found my people. People who, like me, had

worked through much of their own traumatic past and were determined to help minimize the same dysfunction in others. This community led me to complete the TBRI Practitioner Training and introduced me to Karyn's Army, a vast network of caring professionals who use TBRI to try and better the lives of children who have experienced adversity. Over the next few years, I was invited to speak to prospective TBRI Practitioners about the sensory system. I met compassionate, inspiring people who connected me with other professionals working to help children who have experienced adversity. These professionals sent me referrals for their toughest cases, ones many OTs had worked with but could not decipher. These were often children with maladaptive sensory-based behaviors resulting from their trauma histories. I pored through these case studies, eager to provide hope and insight that might help these precious children. I lost sleep. I dreamed of these cases. I googled, prayed, researched, and called in other colleagues.

Nothing compares to the dopamine rush of hearing a caregiver say that something I suggested "finally worked" or led to at least a glimmer of hope. While I wish I could say that I have some sort of magic power or insight, the simple reality is that I'm unafraid to try, and I'm unafraid to fail. I've failed A LOT in my life. I've gained some great stories from those failures — and sometimes I get lucky.

I once worked with a client who had already baffled two pediatricians. I had heard good things about a third pediatrician, who possibly had firsthand experience with this client's condition but was not taking new clients at the time. I delivered a care package of all kinds of goodies to his office. Having worked in medical offices through my high school years, and being related to several physicians, I knew a little gift for the front office staff might help, and certainly couldn't hurt. An obvious bribe would be illegal, of course. But I figured that bringing the front desk staff some treats might gain a little specialized communication and allowance for special circumstances. My plan worked, and I got an appointment for my little guy that very week.

Always take the chance! I've reached out to Jimmy Buffett twice for a meeting. The closest I have gotten is a generic shout-out for my fortieth birthday at a concert. Who knows, maybe someone close to him will someday read this book and tell him how awesome I am and he'll invite me to go flying with him. It can't hurt me to make the suggestion, right? One of my greatest regrets in life is that I never invited Robin Williams to dinner. I'm pretty sure there is zero chance he would have accepted my invitation. But the regret is that I will never know. **Take the chance.** If it might help a child, take two chances.

Much of my success as a therapist is because I don't give up and I keep asking questions of people who have skills I lack. I encourage you to try. Then fail. Then find someone who can take your failed vision and help you. A favorite quote from my father is, "Can't hurt. Might help." Many of my therapeutic hunches are simple, ordinary things that are inexpensive and harmless. Try and eat only left-handed (create novel new neural pathways). Move the child to the head of the table (so they feel empowered). Have them sleep in the opposite direction. Listen to this music. Hug them every two hours. These are all things I've suggested that have been game-changers for clients. Couldn't hurt to try them. Some of them help. The ones that don't help still provide data. As my dad says, "Placebos are fifty percent effective when seventy-three percent of statistics are made up." Those seem like good odds to me!

I've also learned that it isn't always me who helps the client. Research shows that just one caring adult can change the trajectory for a child. Earlier in my career, it was my goal to be that one caring adult. After years of working with exhausted parents, I see that maybe I'm not supposed to be that person. Maybe I am supposed to empower the parents to be that person instead. While less exciting and ego-driven, that change has been profound for me. I realized that even if I got amazing, transformational, goal-meeting, insurance-provider-thrilling results in the clinic, it wasn't really a gain if the child still fell apart at home. But...if I empower the adults in their day-to-day lives with the child, a profound difference can be made. Remember, new neural connections are made through patterned and predictable repetitions. What if the caregiver was unknowingly repeating patterns that undid the work from my clinic? How much more effective could my therapy be if I included the caregiver in my treatment sessions, and taught them to carry over my suggestions? How many more therapeutic repetitions could the child then make in my absence?

Over time, I switched my focus from child-directed therapeutic activity to relationship-focused therapeutic activity. I invited the caregivers into the therapy space with me. When I noticed a weakness or delay, such as an inability to cross the midline, I pointed it out to the caregiver (playfully, always careful not to shame or embarrass the child). I discussed things they could do as part of their daily routine to help strengthen a skill or break a compensatory pattern. Instead of being the therapist one to two hours per week, I became a member of the child's team. In schools, OT is considered a "related service." I like to tell OT students that this means we are relatives! We get to be the wise but cool aunt or playful and protective uncle in the family of care providers. We get to look at the child with compassionate eyes that understand the familial history but aren't part of the day-to-day struggle. We have a holistic outside perspective that makes every family reunion way more fun, especially for the kids.

We must look at brain development through the lens of connection and caregiver relationship. For children from severe adverse experiences or trauma, it is often the relationship part that is lacking. Prior to my immersion in the NMT and TBRI world, I viewed this type of trauma as neglect. However, in my mind, that made it seem like there was some sort of willful discard or casting aside of the infant. While this does happen, sometimes it isn't quite so dramatic. Sometimes, it is a caregiver who is overwhelmed themselves. It took several years of my own therapy and self-compassion to realize I fit in this category with my eldest child.

I remember my boss, and one of the most influential

therapists in my life, Ruth Tobias, OTR/L, once giving a pregnant coworker a tip. She said, "You will be an infinitely better parent having been a therapist. And you will be an infinitely better therapist being a parent." At the time, those words cut me deep. Believing I would never be a parent and wanting to be the best therapist, I was even doubtful and angry about what she said. But then, I lived her words some five short and unexpected years later. She was right. This doesn't mean I was less badass than I thought I was. Indeed, I had my own superpowers. I had energy and innocence for one. I had free time to plan, create, and study my clients. I truly felt like they were my kids. What made me better as a therapist was the understanding of how much a parent will second guess themselves. It was understanding how exhausting it is to have a child who is difficult to calm when you are with them for over the typical OT session time of an hour. It was understanding just how much of your own self-worth could be tied into a little person that may not showcase your amazing parenting proficiency at the most opportune times. It was understanding how lengthy and elaborate home programs are useless if the caregiver doesn't have time, energy, or understanding of the purpose of the exercises.

The years of lengthy home programs and complicated exercises ceased once I realized how incredibly impractical they were for my own child. I gave up a lot of my Applied Behavior Analysis tendencies when I started my journey into trauma research. ABA was a theory developed to analyze behavior and create new neural pathways through repetition. The research is solid. Lots of firing and wiring together. But there was no heart in my experience. There was no emotion. There was no connection. There was no carryover. Some of my colleagues say that ABA is moving more towards function as a treatment model. I hope this is true. My experience has been that it is a lot of hand-over-hand repetition of a tedious non-preferred task.

I would frustratingly express how, given enough repetition, a very small task can be taught. But is it worth the intense time investment and client frustration when that task does not translate to functional skills? For example, a client may practice writing their name 100 times over MANY hours of therapy. But that client has no concept of WHERE to sign their name or how to write any other letters. I gave up ABA because I realized how time- and resource-consuming it is. I realized how little joy and true functionality it added to daily life. In my experience, it not only lacked relationship; it hindered it.

Studying Dr. Perry's NMT and better understanding how we effectively access various parts of our brain based upon our level of arousal (how alert or calm we are) changed the way I practiced OT. Where TBRI uses the terms empower, connect, correct, Dr. Perry refers to the sequence of engagement as regulate, relate, and reason. We can't connect and relate until we empower and regulate. I knew how the child's "engine was running," but I didn't consider the profound and fundamental impact that each engine level had on the child's ability to think or on their behaviors. This understanding helped shift my focus from behavior management to the relational approach that leads to lasting behavioral change. It's about skill, not will. If a child's sensory system is sending them into an "alarm" state, no verbal redirection, hand-over-hand assistance, or visual schedule will fix it. We must support the child first to help provide a sense of felt safety and the sensory foundation to complete the activities we present to them. We have to start back at the beginning. And, in the beginning, our foundation is relationship. Even in a cellular anatomical sense, we began our life when two people had a relationship.

MARTI SMITH, OTR/L

CHAPTER 3

SOMATOSENSORY REGULATION

As I shifted my training focus from autism to trauma-informed care, I first had to explain what "somatosensory" and "regulation" meant. I was noticing that different professions were using these terms inconsistently. As a definition, somatosensory refers to sensations that are not localized to a specific body (somatic) region. This involves the touch and proprioception systems that are interpreted in the somatosensory cortex region of the brain and follow the dorsal column-medial lemniscus pathway. However, it is common for people to use the term somatosensory more broadly to describe how our body reacts to any sensation (visual, vestibular, auditory, olfactory, or gustatory). Regulation, by definition, means to adjust or monitor something. We regulate the sugar levels of someone with diabetes to correctly dose insulin. We use a regulator when scuba diving to control the amount of air that enters our bodies from our oxygen tanks. Although the terms "regulated" and "dysregulated" are often used to describe someone who is too alert or too calm for a given situation, they really don't give us adequate information to assess and treat the person's functional arousal levels.

Regulating is a state of monitoring; it is not a state of being. I find it more useful to refer to my clients as calm or alert since those words describe a state of being. Self-regulation, however, is a sound concept and is often the goal of our treatment. **We want our clients to be able to self-monitor their level of calm or alert, and self-adjust that level based on the current context**.

If we look at the term "regulated" as it is frequently used, it seems to mean that a child is calm, as expected in many social situations (school, church, family dinner, etc.). I want to emphasize that if a child is injured, the healthiest and most socially appropriate response would be to make a lot of noise, cry, or run around. I also wouldn't want a child to simply sit still and be very calm if I were trying to sing and dance or celebrate something with them. As humans, we are designed to have a big range of emotions. So, while I'm most often consulted to calm an overly active child, it is important to realize that sometimes we need alerting activities as well, in order to meet social goals of being regulated. My goal is never to simply calm a child. My goal is to help the child know how their body is feeling so that they can have a socially normative response in a variety of types of events or activities. How boring would it be if we never had our super high or super low reactions?

It is this asynchrony and the inability for an older child to self-regulate that warrants occupational therapy intervention. I mention the older child because, developmentally, younger children do not have the capacity to self-regulate. In regard to brain development, it isn't until a child is four to five years old that they can begin to practice self-regulation. It takes until age ten before this skill is more dependably accessible.

Infants and toddlers rely upon the primary caregiver giving them external cues on how they feel. As they develop language and learn to show more physical signs of emotions, the caregiver labels and responds to these emotions. This exchange happens over and over, creating patterned, repetitive, reinforced neural wiring to help them navigate their senses as these foundational parts of the brain develop. Regulation is taught. The capacity to identify, monitor, and adjust levels of activity based on the chemicals the brain emits is learned early through these social exchanges with a loving caregiver. In the absence of this experience, the brain chemistry continues to default to self-protection and children lose the ability to match their arousal level to our social context.

Worry, alarm, and frustration are biological emotions full of chemicals released by our brains to keep us safe on the cellular level. These emotions are healthy and necessary, but sometimes we need to delay our first reactions to get through brief contextual situations. One way we put these feelings on hold is to dissociate. These brief dissociations are necessary to complete high-emotion tasks. For example, if I am driving and a spider falls into my lap, I need to continue focusing on the road until I can safely pull over. While I appear calm on the outside, I'm using healthy dissociation to survive in the moment. But these feelings still must be felt and expressed. Once I have safely navigated off the road, I'm able to jump out of the car, dance around like a toddler at a hip-hop party, and exclaim some choice words that don't make any sense but are all I can conjure up because I've now lost access to my frontal cortex that stores my good adjectives.

A real-life example of losing my good adjectives was when a teenage neighbor, on her cell phone, backed straight into my honking swagger wagon. The next morning, I had an appointment to assess the damage but it was after school drop off. I calmly told my children they needed to climb in through the back for the ride to school. My son looked me dead in the eye and said, "Yes, Mommy," then proceeded to open the smashed door. I lost my ability to find good adjectives, and instead responded with a few choice words that were not kind or even comprehensible to his young, innocent ears. There may have been a mention of, "Well I hope your seatbelt works if that door doesn't close so you don't fly out on the way to school!" Not a parenting moment I would list on my resume, for sure. Thankfully, the door did close and we drove in very tense silence to school.

In the afternoon, I received a call that my son was called into the office at recess for profanity. He called a kid on the playground a "nincompoop." After stuffing down my shame and muffling my laughter, I calmly explained to his little private Christian school that I was REALLY glad that was the word he chose. Because he certainly had a recent, emotionally-charged example of worse terms. It's a good thing we don't have to be perfect to be proficient at parenting!

When we got home, we had a great discussion as to why it is important to learn your vocabulary words and practice using good adjectives. When we have good adjectives that are practiced prior to times of stress, we can better access them when we are flustered. Study your vocabulary words, my children. It's important. Maybe someday my grandchildren will be less traumatized because my children learned good adjectives.

We can also use these sorts of opportunities to ask for forgiveness when the rage is over. This experience turned into a beautiful parenting moment when I assured my children that when we mess up, it doesn't have to be catastrophic. We can express emotions inappropriately and still have repair. We do the best we can without being shamed by imperfection. We can still love people when we are yelling at them.

The difference between verbal abuse and realistic parenting is that the latter leaves room for repair when the emotions calm down, where the former hinges on dismissiveness, non-accountability, and gaslighting. Admitting we were wrong, expressing remorse for it, acknowledging hurt, and expressing our intent to do better next time is repair. We repair and teach through modeling that to be human means we will sometimes lose control.

The goal is not to avoid feeling things this intensely. My son was only eight years old. It was developmentally appropriate for him to lose focus and fall back on habit during our morning routine. It was equally appropriate for me to be really upset about my busy and already inconvenienced schedule being interrupted. **Big feelings are normal, and their expression keeps us physically healthy. The goal is to be able to express these big feelings in socially appropriate ways and seek repair when they hurt others.**

CHAPTER 4

SENSORY PREFERENCES, NEURAL PATHWAYS, AND CRITICAL WINDOWS OF DEVELOPMENT

My father loves to race cars. For some of my siblings, this was a very relationally positive experience and they themselves love to be at the race track with their own children. I, on the other hand, have some moderate tactile and auditory defensiveness. The loud engines and grit of the dirt in my bed from getting home late was too much for me. When I look at my developmental history, my mother gave birth to me during an incredibly stressful time for her. She was doing the best she could to hold her life together and figure out how she was going to recover from an imminent divorce. There probably wasn't a lot of gazing into my eyes and caressing me. So, my tactile system didn't get the patterned exposure needed for me to be okay with a light touch like a dirt race track or sandy beach. I didn't have normal tactile development.

What is "normal" sensory development? When Dr. Perry talks about normal development, he speaks of making synapses and eventual neural connections through patterned and repetitive action. I love the example another OT gave me once of cows in a pasture. Cows will walk towards water and food. They are heavy enough to make a trail through the grass and vegetation in a pasture. The first few times the cow wanders over to the food, the trail is faint. However, as more cows follow in line and make the journey repeatedly, the grass begins to erode and the path becomes distinct. It becomes so distinct that when a new cow comes into the pasture, they will likely follow the existing path to the water source from the very beginning. It is interesting to note that there have been observed instances where the cows had to walk around an obstacle such as a broken-down tractor or old barn. When the obstacle was removed, the cows continued to follow the well beaten path, even

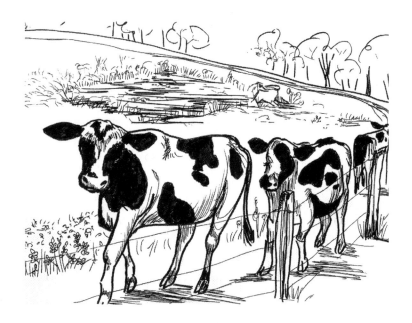

though it would be faster to go directly over the now clear area where the obstacle once stood.

We may think of our neural pathways in a similar fashion. Each time we have an experience, action, event, sensation, or thought, we create electrical and chemical impulses that connect cell nucleus to axon-to-axon terminals, to dendrites, to another cell body. When this happens repeatedly, the portion of the axon called a myelin sheath gets thicker. You can think of myelin like a garden hose. The thicker the hose, the more efficiently the water will flow. If the hose has holes in it, then the water might spill out and your garden will not get the nutrients it needs as quickly. So, you might have to turn up the intensity of the hose. Or you will have to water more often. A nice thick hose means efficient watering. Likewise, a nice thick myelin sheath means efficient neural pathways.

Interestingly, omega fatty acids help form myelin, which is one reason why pregnant women are supposed to take omegas. It is also why nutrition is so important in brain function and explains how poor nutrition (from neglect, picky eating, poverty) can impact sensory preferences and overall brain development. We will look at this a little more when we discuss nutrition in later chapters.

Our cow and garden hose analogies help explain how someone who experienced early adverse experiences may have different brain wiring from someone who grew up without these adverse experiences. As infants, we are completely dependent upon caregivers to keep us safe and form these neuroconnections. It is the caregiver who decides how/when/where to feed us, change our diapers, and look into our eyes. Infants experience a large quantity of painful stimuli as they exit the comfy, temperature-perfect environment of the womb, where their needs are met. Once born, when the infant feels hunger, it is the caregiver who feeds them. They feel better when full. Even in this little interaction, there is a relationship, and that garden hose thickens. Food is one of our first exposures to connection with our caregivers.

The infant's range of vision is only about ten inches. For most women, this is the distance between the nipple and the infant's eyes as they face each other. The hormone that allows the milk to let down is oxytocin, the bonding and love hormone. A similar exchange can happen with bottle feeding and times we engage in a loving interaction. It is important to consider how propping a bottle up as the baby faces away from the caregiver or covering the infant with a nursing blanket inhibits this visual interaction between the child and the caregiver. But when a caregiver holds the infant in the same spot with a bottle, the infant receives much of the same input. The infant learns through repetition that when he is hungry, the mother coos, makes eye contact, chemically connects with, and feeds him. If you've ever watched a caregiver feed an infant, there is often a soft singing, humming (rhythmic vibration), and sometimes even a light touch caress. The light touch should be an alerting sense that would signal danger. But, as the caregiver pairs the relational and rhythmic vibrational sensations for the duration of the feeding, the infant learns that light touch caress signals can be overridden by the rich connective calming influences.

Imagine how many times an infant is fed. That is a lot of repetition and exposure to build those strong neural connections—our garden hose—of "felt safety." Feelings of "It's OK to be alerted by light touch. I can experience pain paired with pleasure and not feel afraid." When we think about the daily life of an infant, we can see many sensory experiences where normal caregiving consists of over-arousal alert activity paired with calming feel-good activity. For example, think about a diaper change. It's uncomfortable at first. It might be cold as the cool air hits the wet bum. There could be pain from a diaper rash. Most caregivers don't simply replace the diaper and set the infant aside. The satisfaction and reward of a fresh, clean baby entices the caregiver to snuggle the baby close in a warm deep touch embrace. Maybe even add a bit of a rhythmic tap on the bum as we dance or bounce a little to bring the infant back to calm...through relationship.

As I help caregivers think through the daily sensory experiences of their newborn, I encourage them to see how we are meant to have unpleasant experiences. Indeed, it helps us to have the paired experience of being uncomfortable, and then being helped to find comfort again. The expression, "what fires together wires together" applies here. As we grow, this pairing helps us to experience unpleasant sensations and know that we will be okay. This is resilience! We acquire it through patterned, predictable adversity followed by comfort from people who love us.

As we consider child development, another key concept to understand is that of "critical windows of development." Human development happens in predictable stages and involves multiple systems. When a learning experience relates to the part of the brain that is developing in that moment, we have hit the "critical window of development," and learning proceeds easily. It is as if a window opens up where all the brain development aligns in unison and it is easiest to teach that growth skill.

As an OT school project, I researched as many developmental charts as I could find and compared, contrasted, and organized them. An underlying principle running through all of them was that, in simplistic terms, the brain develops from the inside out and from back to front. Much of early infant development hinges on vision, which is seated in the back of the brain. How amazing is that?! Attachment theory emphasizes the importance of eye contact while feeding an infant. Infants and toddlers rely upon eye contact with an adult to help ensure that their needs will be met. They don't yet need mathematical concepts or independent problem solving, which are housed in the front of the brain. The critical window of development for vision is infancy.

The critical window of development for sensorimotor exploration is in the toddler years. Toddlers move quickly. Their bones are soft and bendy. Moving, jumping, crashing, and exploring are perfect at this stage. Toddlers don't weigh a lot so when they fall, little damage is done. As the child develops, the critical window of development moves forward from vision to sensory motor and then finally to problem solving in the elementary years.

Muscle development, brain-initiated motor coordination, cognitive understanding of letters, visual acuity, and spatial awareness all open up around age six. Most four-year-olds do not have the strength or dexterity in their finger joints to stabilize and move a pencil. Rather than using their fingers, they end up grasping the pencil too tight in the palm of their hand. These early repeated stroke practices lead to poor grasp patterns going forward, even after the child has developed the muscle strength and dexterity to hold the pencil more efficiently. Referring back to the cow and pasture example, just as the cows continue to follow the path around the newly removed obstacle, a child continues to use the neural pathway that was repeated before their window opened. If we could simply wait until a child is six years old to teach them to write their name (after focusing on hand strengthening playdough, letter recognition, etc. when they are four to five), most children would pick this skill up quickly and easily. However, as many school OTs will lament, we now see preschools putting pencils in toddlers' hands. In their attempt to be academically advanced, they make writing more difficult and create bad habits.

Working within critical windows of development would mean fewer bad motor habits to undo. Playing with playdough and making mud pies in preschool would lead to better pencil grasp patterns in second grade, the grade where we see the most handwriting referrals. But by second grade, the window has closed and those pathways are very strong and difficult to break. Too often, school curriculum is not based on human development and does not incorporate realistic, developmentally appropriate goals and activities for our children. Our children are taught   that they are failures, and they end up working really hard to overcome strong dysfunctional pathways pushed upon them by caregivers. These are not connected, empowering pathways that build foundations for later success. They are pathways we have to spend time correcting, at the expense of time for forming new, positive ones.

We must roll over before we can crawl. We *should* crawl before we walk. We form our lips to say "Mama" before we eat mushy foods that require our lips to close and swallow. I am awestruck and fascinated by human development. How many of the children we work with miss these windows? How many of them are developing bad habits trying to meet expectations that they aren't ready for? How many of them simply don't get the necessary stimulation while the window is open?

One final key to my own understanding of the critical window of development was learning that we are born with the majority of our neurons in our brains. It was only recently that scientists discovered we actually do make new neurons, but as of this writing, the number of new neurons formed after birth is insignificant. When I think of this concept, I like to think of the billions of little neurons wearing running shoes with little headsets. They are simply waiting for the neurochemical commands to tell them where to land in the more frontal parts of the brain. As developmental experiences unfold and repeat, more little neurons run forward. This is where some say the brain is "plastic" when we are younger. We have billions of neurons at the ready. The period of growth from birth to eighteen months 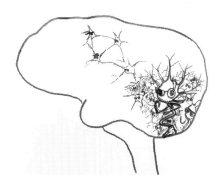 sends eight times more little runner neurons than after age three. Simply put, once we hit age three, many of the runners have hit their landing positions. They are no longer available to run to create new pathways.

I've worked with many children who had a brain injury or a stroke and fully recover, as if it never happened. The child had enough new neurons to create new pathways separate from the ones that were damaged. However, when an adult has a stroke or brain injury, the neurons have all hit their marks and there is a loss of ability to create the new pathways. This is one of the reasons birth-to-three programs do, and should, receive so much government funding. When we can rehab the brain early, there are a lot of runners available to make new, healthy connections.

Another interesting phenomenon about neural connections is that if there is high emotion tied to the experience, the body releases chemicals to make the memory of the experience stronger, which supports increased repetition or avoidance of that action in the future. Thinking of our cow example, the impact of high emotion would be like bringing a lawn mower into our field to make a path for all the cows. While the lawn mower only makes one pass, it leaves a clear path for the cows (neurons) to follow later. This is easy to understand as we think about high emotion experiences of our own. Have you ever choked on a food or gotten violently ill after consuming something you previously enjoyed? If so, you can easily relate to this idea. You may now associate that food with being ill and emphatically avoid it, even if it was previously one of your favorite foods.

Our other senses can also help form these strong pathways. I once was the first person on the scene at a fatal accident. I tried desperately to administer CPR to the man who had (I later found out) suffered a heart attack and hit a tree head on. I can close my eyes and vividly see the scene of the accident. My heart even races a bit as I type this. As I approached the scene, my adrenaline was in overdrive and there was a neural lawnmower in the back of my brain mowing down paths for me to not have to feel this way again. The smell of antifreeze was dense as I straddled him doing compressions until the ambulance arrived. The smell of antifreeze can still take me directly back to that scene as if I'm in a very vivid movie flashback. But it's only the antifreeze that does it. I can see trees. I can see white trucks. I can hear ambulances and interact with men in their fifties without experiencing an elevated heart rate. But the scent of antifreeze was the novel sense in that scene. I already had pathways for men in their fifties, white trucks, and trees.

With our children from trauma, sometimes it is difficult to identify what those lawnmowers could be. It takes a lot of patience, documentation, and discussion to figure out the specific trigger. Sometimes we never can tell what it is. Even without knowing, we must have compassion that those unexplainable triggers are strong. Those lawnmower emotions are very real and compelling for the children we work with.

It is important to highlight how smell is a sense that connects directly to the amygdala, the part of the brain responsible for strong memories. Smell does not go through the thalamus like other sensory input. In early times, a keen sense of smell was vital to our survival. Our brains are very adaptive and strong memories are often tied to smell. Each person has a unique smell and culturally, we are very connected to our heritage through smell. My grandma made the best sugar and molasses cookies. The smell of vanilla or cinnamon transports me back to happy family gatherings and her sweet cookies. In Austin, there are many families whose heritage includes curry. Being a girl from the Midwest, I was conditioned by my family to consider table pepper spicy. When I was older and my husband and I were looking for a new home, I would immediately rule out the ones that smelled of curry. Curry wasn't part of my heritage. I had no experience with it, so it wasn't a positive preference for me.

I'm pleased to say that my friend group has since widened ethnically. I don't exactly seek or prefer the smell of curry, but I no longer have quick reactions of distaste to it. But it took **relationships** with people who love curry for that to happen. I don't feel like it is my place to speak on racism as a blonde, white female. But I can speak to brain science. If we have no relational familiarity to sensory experiences, we will first react with fear. I am frustrated by the phrase, "We aren't born racist." Because, in a way, we are. Our early life experiences build those implicit bias pathways based on experience. We have genetic imprints to seek care from those who look and smell similar to us. Genetically speaking, the best way to combat racism is positive early exposure to diversity. Children need to develop those congruent learning pathways together. Pathways where there is an element of "Oh...that seems scary, I don't have a reference for that," paired with "My caregiver is in relationship with me and I can follow their cues that I am safe." Eventually, with enough paired exposures like this, the child is able to form their own preferences for what is safe and familiar. Maybe these preferences will even mean that my white children will like curry.

This is important to understand because caregivers who interact with children from trauma might have a different color skin than the child. They may be unfamiliar. They may be biologically perceived as a threat. It is only through repeated positive pairing relationships that these new connections, perceptions, and preferences are made. The opportunity to increase a child's sense of safety is just one reason why it is imperative to include people of diverse backgrounds when we look at staffing and authority figures who will be interacting with children.

My colleague Robyn Gobbel, LCSW, LMSW, RPT-S, highlights the idea that our self-perception is reflected in our caregivers. This perception begins very early in development with the mirror neurons. When we make faces and coo at a baby, remembering that vision and attachment are the infant's current "Critical Window of Development," we send the message to the child that they are "seen." We want to be like them, and thus they want to be like us. We copy infants instinctively. Through seeing us, we teach them about themselves.

Infants have not yet developed autonomy and therefore they learn who THEY are through their caregivers' reflection. When my infant was trying to eat and my eyes, heart rate, posture, and tone reflected frustration to her, she learned that she was a source of frustration. Even typing this sentence grieves me. I write with hope that someone will read it and take it to heart while their baby is still in that developmental window, and that my failing will help prevent that trauma for another precious baby who is struggling to eat. I also type this with hope and insight on repair. My child and I have worked very hard to re-attach later in life. I now have the life experience to know there is no perfect parent. But as long as we can strive for honest connection and unconditional love when we know better, there is hope for future relationships.

Dr. Perry once described brain development in terms of H20. An infant brain is like vapor. A simple puff of air can change the course of the molecules. When we have early intervention, the changes seem to require less effort and less repetition. There are simply more neurons to influence. As the brain develops and a child enters the preschool years, the brain is more like water. We can still influence and change the course, but there will be more back pedaling and resistance. Change isn't as quick or effortless. The adolescent and adult brains are more like ice. Changing the course for a more developed brain is like chipping away at an ice sculpture. It takes a lot of repetition, patience, skill, and perseverance. Change is always possible. But it is important to keep our expectations realistic and understand what we are capable of influencing.

My friend and colleague, Michael Remole, gave me another helpful analogy about brain functioning. He describes the child's body as a bus and the brain as the driver. Who is driving the bus? Is it the emotional Limbic Larry? Or is it thoughtful Cortex Charlie? For some of the children we work with, Limbic Larry hijacks the bus and it's already headed for a busy intersection before Cortex Charlie can stop it. Sometimes we can do all the "right" things therapeutically and still crash that bus. But if we can toss some barricades in the road (compassionate support systems), there is still hope of the bus not breaking apart or hurting others.

My aunt worked in child welfare group homes in the 1970s and '80s, and she once passed along a story to me that I have since shared many times over. It has made an impact on my teaching and my insistence that every life is worthy of our efforts. Sometimes our expectations simply need to be better suited to match the ability of the children we work with. The story is about a case meeting where the staff was overwhelmed, and one particular child seemed like a lost cause. In the best Texas drawl I can imagine, the administrator calmly stood up and proclaimed, "Whelll…I can say we probably can't stop him from robbin' the convenience store. But I sure as hell hope we can prevent him from killin' the clerk."

This story reminds me of many children I've worked with, who have so much experience with trauma that their pathways are wired for survival instead of connection. Many of them WILL be repeat offenders. It would be unrealistic to think that if we were just all "trauma informed," there would be no more crime, and we could all sing around campfires together. BUT, what an impact even the smallest hope of connection and humanity could bring. What if the work we put in and invest in these children doesn't create valedictorians, but maybe they can hold a steady job as a vet tech? Maybe they still engage in petty crime because they will always have food insecurity. But they do so in nonviolent ways. I know the family of that convenience store clerk will be VERY glad we didn't give up on that child.

This story highlights another way that development can be less than ideal. This child maybe didn't have the best models for how to get his needs met. When children are neglected, they often don't have good relationally paired associations and pathways. They simply don't have any experience that tells them what is socially expected of them.

How can we expect a child who has never experienced respect to be respectful? If a person is struggling to swim, we don't shame them and yell at them to do the breaststroke. We first bring them to safety and then teach them swim skills that will prevent a future drowning. The child must feel safe to learn. Our expectations must match the child's learned or missed experiences. Our expectations must match the child's ability. We start with a doggy paddle.

Children who are exposed to violence, unpredictability, and other intense sensations have learned that the world can hurt them. Studies show that in these children, the amygdala (memory and activation of fear response) is larger in size compared to age-related norms. These children often have many lawnmowers in their brain making large protective pathways. While they can appear to be very controlling and dominating, they are simply trying to stay alive in the only way they know how. They have learned that so many things are harmful to them. This is their truth. This is their lived experience. This is why they are often hypervigilant and appear over-alert.

Intense sensation can come from the kind of physical trauma we associate with police shows or dramatic documentaries. But it could also be from necessary medical trauma. The skin is one of the first sensory organs to develop outside of the womb. From the first puff of air upon delivery, the skin helps the infant understand their environment and how it relates to themselves and their need for warmth, connection, and protection. When a child has early medical intervention, often the skin is poked, prodded, stuck, and adhered to. In the early 1980s, Patricia Wilbarger, MEd, OTR, FAOTA, identified premature infants developing what OTs call tactile defensiveness, from all the tubes and sensors being taped to them. Because of her work, NICUs now encourage skin-to-skin contact with caregivers. We use less noxious or invasive ways to attach sensors and sticky things that would otherwise flood the brain with adverse tactile input.

After studying the neuroscience of how pathways are made, I started to see how **relationship** was a missing piece to my therapy sessions. I have a natural ability to connect and build rapport. But I wasn't helping the caregiver carry over that rapport with the child. I was great at working on oral motor skills and helping the child latch onto a bottle and meet feeding goals. But feeding my own child was a very different story.

My active lifestyle and "inability to have kids" led me to a breast reduction in my early twenties. Since I believed I was infertile, I told the surgeon to not be concerned with saving the milk ducts. I wouldn't need them. Oh, how wrong I was. I could probably write an entire comical and heart-wrenching book about breastfeeding post-reduction.

In 2005, my social network was ALL about breastfeeding. I felt like a complete failure and worried that my baby would not have the neurotransmitters (remember oxytocin), immunity, nutrition, etc., if I couldn't produce milk. I tried every trick I could find. I exhausted myself trying to produce just a few ounces. I remember one comically tragic moment when I spent nearly two hours pumping only two ounces of precious breast milk. I tripped walking into the kitchen and those little plastic vials went sailing through the air and pathetically spilt onto my tile floor in seemingly slow motion. I burst into a hormonal downpour of tears. My sweet husband walked in, saw what happened, wrapped his arms around me and compassionately whispered, "In this case, it's okay to cry over spilled milk."

My meltdown had very little to do with the actual milk. It had more to do with the feelings that milk represented. Feeding an infant is a BIG deal, and nothing I knew about brain chemistry or physical development prepared me for the failure I felt at not being able to provide food for my child. Food is a basic need. It is a biological longing within us to show love through food. When someone has a tragedy, we bring food. When we gather, we have food rituals and special dishes. We eat comfort food for its emotional value. When I couldn't help my child eat, I felt a deep sense of failure. While I focused on the physical aspects of feeding my infant, I missed some very important connection and relationship aspects.

As my child is now preparing to launch into her adult world, I sometimes long to go back and have a redo of our first years before I found TBRI and the NMT. But I realize that the power of reconciliation is strong. I wouldn't have the energy of my early thirties. I love a meme I saw once that read, "I will give you love, nurture, and just enough dysfunction to make you interesting." Oh, how I have clung to that. Interesting dysfunction aside, Suzy and I have worked to overcome those early years of "misattunement." We have learned to give each other space when emotions need to be expressed. We recognize and validate when the other person simply needs to be heard and not helped. We make attempts to hold off on emotional conversations until we are fed and rested. I don't force her to eat meat and she cooks soups to share without as much spice as she would like to add. I appreciate our relationship and time together more each year. She tells me (as a teenager) that she loves me. That seems pretty significant. I think we did our best with what we were given and we will continue to do better as we know better.

When we view sensory development through the lens of trauma, it is important to understand, once again, the value of the loving caregiver connection and relationship. Not all sensory input is equal. Our sensory preferences are greatly shaped by our lived experiences. Take this scenario for example. A caregiver is playfully wrestling with a child and accidentally knocks them in the eye with an elbow. The caregiver immediately recognizes what happens, swoops the child up, provides that calming/pain-overriding deep touch input, and renders aid to the child. The child has learned that pain isn't to be feared. Even though the injury was caused by the caregiver, the child does not perceive the caregiver as unsafe. This child develops resilience and remains connected.

While consulting with Dr. David Cross in regard to a TBRI project, he suggested I use a chart format to help describe how trauma affects the developing sensory systems. As most of his suggestions are, it was brilliant. This chart helps the reader understand a little more about the Critical Windows of Development and how trauma may

WHAT IS DEVELOPING?					
In Utero	Birth	0-2 months	2-36 months	3-6 years	6-12 years
Vestibular system and neural tube forming	Oxytocin and attachment hormones and proprioception, O2 stats	Vision and visual processing, arousal and survival rhythms	Speech, language, and hearing	Sensory Motor systems	Reasoning, planning, organizing, personality, memory, empathy, relationships

HOW DEVELOPMENT IS DISRUPTED					
In Utero	Birth	0-2 months	2-36 months	3-6 years	6-12 years
Maternal movement, substance use, and nutrition are incredibly influential during this period	Birth trauma can impact attachment, ability to stimulate the proprioceptive system, and feeding, ICU can assault the tactile system	Much of the 0-2 month old is about seeing, feeling, and smelling the caregiver. Lots of sleep/wake/feed cycles that form attachment and the ability to self-soothe through repeated caregiver guidance	Language acquisition may be delayed with neglect, hearing sensitivities with chaotic environments	Large muscles are beginning to form and become coordinated for walking, crawling, hopping, running, balance, and crossing midline	A chaotic or unorganized environment can hinder organization, planning, and reasoning. Routine, consistency, and modeling are big influences during this time.

HOW THE OLDER CHILD MIGHT PRESENT					
In Utero	Birth	0-2 months	2-36 months	3-6 years	6-12 years
May notice: poor balance, poor wake/sleep cycles,	Loud and rapid talkers because they can't catch a full breath, poor proprioceptive function from not going through the birth canal, attachment issues	Feeding difficulty, sleep difficulty, difficulty scanning the environment, later difficult with reading	Poor speech patterns, difficulty with language and auditory processing	Poor balance, difficulty crossing the midline of the body, tactile sensitivity, poor coordination	Disorganized, impulsive, need for control, untrusting, explosive, lethargic and unengaged

influence those neural connections during the maturity of the structures responsible for sensory processing.

In the NMT teaching, Dr. Perry gives much consideration to the impact of trauma on the different parts of the developing brain. One of the core principles of this model is that the brain develops in a predictable sequence and must be rehabbed in a similar predictable sequence. As an occupational therapist, I could really grasp this concept. After all, I had studied and worked in outpatient rehab for about a decade on the side of my full-time school therapy job.

I was well aware of, and comfortable with, doing an activity analysis to determine where the "hitch in the giddyup" could be found. If a person lost motion of the arm, we started the rehab at the shoulder. It doesn't make sense to work on fingers before you have trunk stability. I had a thorough understanding of the need for a strong base of support (proximal stability) before skilled movement of the extremities (distal mobility). Therefore when Dr. Perry started talking about brain stem foundations and hierarchy heuristics, these concepts were easy for me to relate to. Oh, the irony of learning about repeated exposures and learning and brain changes while I'm receiving these repeated exposures.

It is helpful to understand that these brain development hierarchy skills build upon one another. If a child doesn't have good eye control, they will struggle with reading and math because their eye muscles will not move in the smooth pursuits to interpret the words or numbers. This was not new information for me. But the organization of the information in the NMT caused it to "click" as I began to see my clients through the lens of adverse life events and how they would later impact development. It was a way for me to better work my way backwards in my activity analysis of the chain of events that led to the behavior or skill I was addressing in my therapeutic goals. When I added the TBRI filter to the NMT lens, it was as if I could more clearly see these therapeutic goals/targets through relationships.

Having not had a relationship-rich childhood to build my own neural connections of understanding and compassion, gaining understanding of how relationship is foundational to early neural experiences was profound for me. As I considered that many therapists come from high ACE scores themselves, it became the motivation for me to write this book. I want others to better see the biological basis behind some of the skills the children we serve are lacking. In later chapters, I will address some remediation or rehabilitative activities that move those children forward in their own neurological growth. But in order to understand what part of the process/activity is causing the dysfunction, we need to clearly understand all of the parts to that process/activity. Occupational therapists spend years studying activity analysis. Our training makes us specialists in breaking down tasks into minute steps. This makes us expert problem solvers and sets us apart from other rehabilitation professionals. **Our unique expertise is why I strongly advocate for an occupational therapist to be on the trauma team.**

CHAPTER 5
CALMING OR ALERTING?

One of my teaching handouts that I am often asked to copy is a calming versus alerting list. I first created this list while working with children with autism. After hearing from teachers who wanted to help decrease aggressive and self-harm behaviors in the classroom, I put on my sensory detector lenses and tried to help them think through ways the environment might be unintentionally alerting the child. While I will share that handout in this book, I want to be clear about its limitations, the most significant being that it is not universally applicable to all people. Not only are we uniquely and wonderfully made, we have different life experiences. Our genetics, life experiences, and specific relational cues *combined* are what make up our sensory preferences. I used the example of smelling like monkeys in the first chapter. I'm guessing not many others have that same sensory preference. I know my classmate definitely did not.

It is unreasonable to think we are all identical or will react identically to the same stimuli. We don't all have the same heritage, genetic makeup, or life experiences. So, it is through this lens that I forge forward with sensory tips and suggestions. It is important to understand that the preferences and tendencies I discuss are just that—tendencies. It is expected that some of these strategies will not work for some individuals. As my father says, they "can't hurt, might help." I am confident you can use them without causing harm. They are worth trying. What a boring world it would be if we all had the same sensory preferences. How would we even grow? Who would introduce this midwestern girl to spices like curry? We grow best when pushed outside of our comfort zones within supportive relationships. I hope that whatever strategies you do attempt are done within the context of connection and relationship.

When we discuss sensory preferences, we can observe generalized patterns of activities that calm and activities that alert. Keep in mind, though, that these ideas are not prescriptive but rather, researched or probable suggestions. One of the most frequent requests I get as an occupational therapist is for help "regulating a child." I accomplish this often through the lens of what activities are alerting versus calming, which I have outlined in this handy little chart:

TACTILE

Considerations	Tips to Calm	Tips to Alert
Light touch is the threat response	Soft, consistent textures	Uneven/Inconsistent textures
Deep touch is the thought response	Minky blankets	Feathers
First to develop in utero	Weighted blankets (SmartWeight)	Tickles
Easy to access or insult	Firm pressure/rubs	Light pressure
Increased sensitivity on hands, face, feet, and genitalia	Tight clothing	Cold
Shuts down when overstimulated	Heavy clothing	One handed touch
Stimulation can last up to two hours	Warmth	Movement from the base of the spinal cord towards the head
	Two-handed touch	
	Movement from the base of the neck towards the bottom of the spinal cord	

VISION

Considerations	Tips to Calm	Tips to Alert
The peripheral/side vision is the threat response	Blues, greens, and browns	Yellows, reds, and oranges
The focal/midline vision is the thought response	Linear lineups	Circular or chaotic lineups
Infant field of vision is only 10-12 inches, it is easily overstimulated with outward facing carriers	Looking up	Peripheral stimulation
Eye muscles develop in coordination with crawling, something many children from trauma do not do	Rhythmic side to side eye movement	
Over-scanning in childhood can make the visual system over-reactive	Focal/midline concentration	
Eyes are connected directly to the vestibular system and help to "stabilize" the vestibular system	Moving into a room with brighter light	
(spotting when spinning)	Wearing a ball cap (a "blinder" for horses)	
Pupils are responsive to stress		

AUDITORY

Considerations	Tips to Calm	Tips to Alert
Music is multi-sensory as it pulls in vibration (proprioception)	50-70 BPM like early Mozart	90-120 BPM like Lady Gaga
-	-	-
Fluid from frequent ear infections can cause hearing processing issues	Familiar melodies	Unfamiliar melodies
-	-	-
Different frequencies are heard differently	Habituated sounds	Arrhythmic patterned sounds
-	-	-
Sound vibrations can adjust the heart rate and therefore alert status	Patterned humming	Arrhythmic drumming
-	-	
Sound can be very culturally relevant	Rhythmic drumming	
-		
Singing and speaking are processed in different brain regions		
Sound can be conducted via bones		
-		
Music can be a simple external influence		

SMELL

Considerations	Tips to Calm	Tips to Alert
Assists with taste	Vanilla	Smoke
-	-	-
Very primitive	Cinnamon	Musk
-	-	-
Direct access to the emotion centers	Sugar	Onion
-	-	-
Often alerts the fight/flight/freeze response	Flour	Floral
-	-	-
Forms strong neural connections to memories	Pleasing (individual preference) smells	Peppermint
-	-	-
Cultural and familial ties	Familial smells	A smell associated with a traumatic experience or event
	-	
	Lavender	

56

TASTE		
Considerations	**Tips to Calm**	**Tips to Alert**
Food is one of our first biological needs and is met in our first caregiver relationships	Sweet	Spicy/peppermint
-	-	-
For many, food = love, acceptance, safety, needs met	Chewy (proprioception)	Foods that scatter in the mouth
-	-	-
To deny food is to deny life	Sucking/midline pulling like straws, biting nails, and smoking	Licking
-	-	-
Food is highly relational	Warm foods	Cold
-	-	-
Adverse childhood events can influence oral motor abilities (tongue might not move correctly and the child feels like they are choking easily)	Culturally comforting foods	New/unfamiliar foods
-		
Caregiver guilt when a child rejects food		
-		
Food /nutrition influence cell structure		
-		
Dehydration causes electrolyte imbalance - literal brain chemistry		
-		
Food is a large influence of culture and familial structure		
-		
Taste and smell are heavily connected. If you freeze food, it doesn't smell. Some children are more likely to eat food without an overpowering smell.		

Before I go further into sensory experiences, I want to revisit the word "regulation" as defined in Chapter 3. Most times, when someone refers to a child as "dysregulated," they are simply stating that the child's level of activity does not match the social environment. We can't regulate a person. What we can do is increase or decrease their arousal level. We can influence them internally or externally to calm or alert them. They can then use self-regulation to monitor whether or not their activity/arousal level matches the social environment and circumstance. While the term "co-regulate" is often used as a description of a caregiver monitoring and influencing the arousal/activity level of both themselves and the child, a better description would be to say the caregiver is mirroring, relating, influencing, and joining the child in calming or alerting activity. An important reminder from Chapter 3 as we consider ways to influence a child's arousal level is that the goal is not always to calm, but rather to match the social context.

How do we teach self-regulation? How does a child learn to monitor their own level of activity/arousal? In short, they learn it through the eyes of a connected caregiver. Most infant responses are reflexive. When the caregiver matches the level of energy/arousal that a reflex initiates, the child feels "seen" and learns how to interpret sensory input and how those feelings fit into the social world. The caregiver's tone, heart rate, facial expression, and tempo/rhythm mirror the child's reflexive responses and lead the child (through connection, communication, and relationship) into the state of arousal that fits the moment. Trauma impacts this learning, since the child's needs are not met within the normal social framework.

When a child's cries are not met with movement, empathy, or urgency, there is no pathway created to reinforce a base of co-regulation—that ability to match an arousal state with a connected caregiver. Some neglected children learn to simply not cry. They no longer "feel" but instead dissociate. They may become apathetic and show little awareness of self-care as they get older. They become avoidant. Alternatively, a neglected infant may become inconsolable, as if signaling endlessly to a caregiver who doesn't respond. Without learning how to interpret their own sensory experiences, they may seek more sensory input to try and have more data points to understand what is happening in their bodies. They appear hyperactive or "sensory seeking."

Other children have caregivers who respond inconsistently to those reflexive sensory cues. These children form pathways that are scattered, disorganized, and unpredictable. No one path becomes dependably myelinated. These children become difficult to calm. They simply don't have the experience of the repeated calming that is required to learn. Their ability to monitor their arousal state or self-regulate is not developed because they simply haven't had consistent repeated neural firing to develop this skill. Their behaviors become inconsistent as well. One minute they are seeking sensory input and the next, sensations become overwhelming, often with very little warning.

As a therapist, I first recognize that the child's inability to monitor and adjust their arousal level is not intentional. I appreciate how Dr. Stuart Ablon discusses will versus skill. He says children do well when they can. It's not that they want to fail. They need Dr. Perry's six Rs of sensory learning: Rhythmic Repetition in the context of a Relationship that is Relevant, Rewarding, and Respectful. It is exhausting to have no foundation or awareness of sensory interpretation.

Babies need a caregiver who introduces them to squishy food and makes noises with their lips, mirroring the lip movement needed to accept the food. They need a caregiver who puts words to their feelings, internal and external, emotional and physical. Babies need a caregiver who helps them move from discomfort back to comfort, thousands of times per day, through connection, compassion, and consistency. In trauma, these early learning experiences simply don't happen—or worse, are harmful. Dr. Purvis points out that a child who is hurt in relationship can only come to healing through healthy relationship. When the person who was supposed to cherish and protect you harms you, it is difficult to trust and receive the repeated positive experience for connected neural pathways. Children who are mistreated often push away the very thing that will help them. We must work diligently to find ways to engage with them in ways that feel safe to them. Sometimes this means going backward developmentally. We mirror them. We respond to them by meeting their needs without expectations, as we would with a much younger child. We parallel play with them. We adapt their environment to meet their sensory preferences.

To influence calm or alertness by adapting the environment, we can refer to the chart on pages 67-69. But to use these ideas most effectively, we must understand further how the body responds to stimuli. We must also understand that we learn from extremes, like a pendulum. We might first make a mark on paper that is too dark, then too light. Finally, we figure out what is just right. Our caregivers help us learn which mark is just right through their reaction to each of our failures. We play with language and make many sounds individually and repeatedly before we form words, and later, sentences. Sentences we hear repeated and modeled by those in our social circles. We experiment with loud and quiet before we find conversational volume. We tickle and tackle before we touch moderately.

Sensory learning is similar. We often have to push a child just to the limits of what is comfortable and then slightly further for a very brief duration before we pull them back into their comfort level. The area where they are already comfortable can be called their "window of tolerance." For many children, their window of tolerance is too small. As therapists, our job is to help open that window wider, so that they learn to self-regulate within a wider range of activities.

As I write this chapter, I am teaching my son to ski. Simply renting him skis did not help him swoosh down the mountain. We had to start on the bunny hill. He needed short, successful runs with a little bit of fear to engage the parts of his brain that will help him learn to keep his head off the snow. He needed the just right amount of fear. Too much fear would leave him mentally frozen on the hill. Not enough fear could send him careening through the trees without skill for safety. With each run, his confidence grew steadily as he was able to complete bigger hills and longer runs. With each run, his window of tolerance opened up a bit. It was a gradual process that involved many repetitions and a few falls.

As we boarded a ski lift, I realized just how therapeutic skiing is. My son was terrified the first time he boarded an open lift, so we started with the gondola, an enclosed lift. I met him within his window of tolerance. I validated him. I gave him a taste of how fun going down a little hill could be. I provided a helmet and I stayed by his side for a sense of felt safety. Then, in the context of a relationship, we slowly

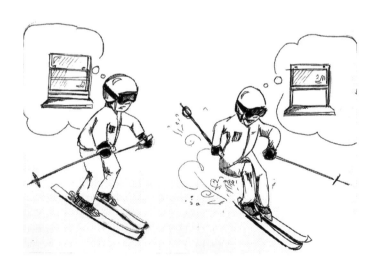

advanced his comfort and skill.

On one particular lift ride, we observed a "skier yard sale." This is a term used when a skier wipes out so forcefully that their gear goes flying everywhere and it looks like they are left amongst a collection of their belongings, like a yard sale. Immediately after, we witnessed this skier's entire group, one by one, make sure she was okay. Some of her party gave her verbal encouragement. Some helped her collect her bargain items. Others stood by and laughed and began the process of creating a narrative about that event.

The narrative wasn't "You have no skill. You fell and embarrassed yourself. You are worthless." The narrative was, "Wow! That looked epic! We asked if you were okay because we care about you. We stopped our activity and fun to make sure you could continue to join us. We want to make sure you know you are part of our group. You were seen. You matter. Let's try that again, together."

A cultural event lost on modern Americans is the after-hunt campfire. Dr. Cross teaches on the importance of verbal storytelling where events are retold, reframed, and the main characters are reaffirmed. I find hobbies like skiing to be the modern hunt where the story is still told around the campfire. For the rest of the lift ride, I imagined that group retelling the story to others in their party that were not present at the event. Retelling that story for years to come, just as my family did for my own epic stories of getting tangled in tree branches in attempts to ski off the trails.

No good story starts with, "I was eating a salad..." or

ends with "...and everything went according to plan." No, our stories — the things that people mirror and reflect to us about who we are — most often deal with adversity and how we overcame it. Often, they involve poor judgement: "Here, hold my beer!" or "I **think** we can make it..." or "Aw, it will be fine!" Maybe they take an unexpected turn: "All of the sudden...". They most often end with a way the event turned out okay in the end. A way someone helped them recover. A way that makes a great story full of excitement, suspense, resolution, and relationship.

I often remind my children that I'm trying to make them interesting, especially after another one of many repairs I have had to have with them because of my personality or a failed attempt at fun. My husband jokes that my tombstone will say, "She tried." He has also instructed the kids to put "He paid for it" on his tombstone. I bought an old RV at the start of the COVID-19 lockdown and he didn't complain about the many costly repairs and tow truck bills that come from owning an old RV. I make elaborate plans for last minute camping and forget to pack the blankets. He figures out how to Amazon Prime them to our campground. I say, "Aw, it will be fine!" as we cross an extremely narrow and wet log over a waterfall. He holds the children with a very strong hand as we cross. I bring shenanigans and adventure to our family, and he brings safety and security. It's a great partnership.

I've spent overnights in an RV stuck in a snowbank. I've rented cars with strangers at an airport during a snowstorm. I've survived a plane crash in Mexico. I've witnessed leaving a sibling at a gas station unknowingly. (We didn't even go back for the sibling. The police took her home, two states away, to our neighbor who watched her for the rest of the week.) While a bit distressing at the time, these are stories my children hear retold through tears of laughter from my siblings. My daughter, who tends towards my husband's sense of safety, once said, "It's better to write a lame story than an obituary." **I would add, "It's good to write a life story with people who balance us."**

I've often wondered what made these childhood stories funny and not debilitatingly traumatic. The common thread is community. As we were stuck in the snowbank or tent without blankets, we huddled together. We encouraged each other. We didn't go through the experience alone. We had a neighbor and several state police officers who cared for the left-behind sibling. She had a loving community that cared for her until our return, a week later. She had compassionate caregivers giving her support and love and confirming her narrative that our family is dysfunctional. But that didn't mean she wasn't loved. The adults around her sent repeated affirming positive narratives to help her not "feel" abandoned, when in fact she literally was. How others reflect our experiences back to us, especially as young children, greatly shapes who we become and how we view ourselves and others. This does not mean that we lie to our children or insist they don't feel the way they are expressing. It means we validate those feelings and help them recognize that they are not alone in them. We offer them a warm beverage and a soft blanket while we listen and reflect with them.

Experience reflection is vital to sensory system development. The development of a tactile narrative, and thus the neural groundwork for tactile sensations of pain, is built within relationships. Consider when a child reaches up and touches a hot stove. With a connected caregiver, the wound is immediately tended to. The caregiver matches the level of distress with a high pitched, "Oh, MY! Are you OKAY? Let me SEE!" Care is given, proprioceptive input is placed over the wound in the form of a bandage or the caregiver's own hand. The pain is stopped (we will explore this further later) through CONNECTION and care. The child learns that the stove is hot and can burn. The child also learns that they can overcome a burn because they had someone walk through the pain with them and provide the care they needed. This child can quickly move on about their day, with little check-ins here and there, and could become a successful chef who loves a good hot stove later in life.

With a caregiver who is not connected, the child receives very different neural firing experiences and groundwork. Maybe the caregiver exploded and blamed the child, causing fear of being yelled at again. Or they find the matched energy to be a comfort and seek it out again and again. They look for things that hurt them because it takes that much input to finally get a reaction, to feel "alive" and "seen," if even in a negative light. They could engage in behaviors such as lying about how the events unfolded to cover up the shame. The process of reconciliation and forgiveness is not modeled, and they are therefore unable to extend those skills to others in the future.

The child who doesn't receive care may learn that stoves, and possibly everything that is red, is scary. This child has no context for how to care for the burn, and the parts of the brain that store memory become overactive to make sure that child doesn't experience that pain again. The child may become "controlling," "manipulative," and many other words we use to describe a child who is trying to avoid experiencing pain. This child learns that no one is looking out for their interest, so it is important that they protect themselves at the cost of relationship to others. If we don't teach children with repetitive examples how to interpret events through our eyes, we can't expect them to know what we are looking for from them in the future.

With a non-connected caregiver, the child does not learn to be part of a community. They lack the framework to understand that adversity can be okay if matched with the care from their community. The popular ACES (Adverse Childhood Experiences) study is a simple checklist that correlates adverse childhood experiences with disease diagnosis and behaviors such as missed work and drug abuse. The adverse experiences being considered in this study (divorce, parental incarceration, abuse, and others) are in the context of relationships. Car accidents, medical birth trauma, burns on a stove or from a fire, and other forms of non-relational traumatic events are less indicative of future disability or behavioral vulnerability. When we look at trauma that encourages community support, we find that there is more resilience. When caregivers lack this community, so do the children.

We can view this relational involvement through Dr. Perry's teaching on resilience versus vulnerability, in which he discusses that many children from adverse experiences develop resilience. On the other hand, we find other children who experience less outright adversity yet become vulnerable and have difficulty with daily activities. When the pattern of stress is unpredictable, extreme, or prolonged, it leads to sensitization and vulnerability. When the pattern of stress is predictable, moderate, and controllable, it leads to tolerance and resilience.

Resilience hinges on a connected caregiver to buffer the pattern of stress for the child.

I have often wondered about the role of resilience in my own family. My nine siblings and I have all grown up into different lifestyles. We are a very blended family, so it is expected that with our various genetics, environments, and life experiences, we would have very different outcomes. What has always surprised me was how, from the early teenage years, two of my eldest siblings seemed to have more vulnerability than others.

I remember once having a conversation with my father about my frustrations with him not being present in my life. I distinctly remember him saying, "Well. At least you know who I am. I think kids (like these two siblings) who grow up not knowing their father do worse."

It is a really interesting memory. I find it fascinating. It seems so true. Many studies show that children who grow up without a father figure become more vulnerable. Studies also demonstrate that society makes it difficult for families who struggle financially to make a marriage work, and that it's almost a better financial arrangement if they aren't together. So much of our welfare system is more damaging than helpful in regard to children knowing their fathers.

Dr. Perry teaches that the outcome is better for a child who experiences more intense, longer-lasting trauma after the age of three than a child who experiences acute trauma in the first two months of life. This has been profound and eye-opening for me. Within my own family, the siblings who have struggled the most with addiction and with maintaining healthy intimate relationships had really rough beginnings. Their fathers abandoned their mothers, and I can imagine these mothers felt they were left without a good support system.

I don't know the exact details and their stories are not mine to tell, but I do know both of these mothers went on to raise subsequent less vulnerable children and I've seen their anguish and love for their daughters who struggle. I find it interesting that I, myself, had a very traumatic start. I don't know all the details of my infancy. These aren't things my mother will discuss openly. But I do know that my mother had already decided to leave my father during her pregnancy and she remarried when I was very young. She did have someone who supported her. I had six older siblings. I had an older sister who was eight at the time I was born and must have thought I was the coolest baby doll ever. She is usually the one holding me in family photos. I had connected caregivers. They may not have been adults, but they met my needs. I had a brother thirteen months older who was my very best friend. The adversity we faced, we faced together.

My older siblings without a father present at their birth did not have those sibling relationships during their infancy. They didn't have siblings who could gaze at them, mirror them, and relate to their experience. My family has a saying that we laugh about and are very fond of. Before setting off on an adventure, "You gotta have a buddy and a helmet." Growing up, there were always motorcycles, race cars, four wheelers, and the like. My father is a big adrenaline seeker who never expected to live past thirty, as his own father died young. Through my entire existence he has lived for the moment. But he also worked in an ER. He knew firsthand that broken bones and such heal pretty easily. But head injuries dramatically decrease your quality of life. So, you could jump off the roof, drive on a sidewalk, swim without an adult in the home, ride motorcycles, and basically run feral through the woods. But if there was a risk of head injury, you better have a helmet on.

Having a buddy was important to later tell the tale to EMS as well as laugh about it during subsequent family gatherings. A buddy and a helmet. Without being a psychological trauma expert, I feel like my dad was wise beyond my own understanding in the 1980s. He knew that relationships and heritage were the greatest buffer against adverse life choices. My family history is riddled with trauma that goes back generations. My dad laughed as he once told me, "You know, some family trees show the members sitting on the branches. Our relatives tended to be the ones hanging from them." I am descended from a long line of large families and storytellers. We have buddies and stories told over a barbecue that buffer the effects of some of our traumatic events.

Dr. Perry's research has also shown that if the adversity is patterned and predictable the chance of vulnerability declines and the chance of resiliency increases. In my own childhood, my siblings and I knew we would be shut in the room together. We knew my brother could sneak out the window, climb on the roof to the kitchen so his footsteps weren't heard, and gather food for us. We had games we would play together to pass the time. The adversity of being locked in a room for extended periods was patterned and predictable.

For some children, they know when the caregiver comes home drunk, there will be physical or sexual abuse. Many of these children will instigate the abuse so that they can have control of the timing. They create this predictability based on the pattern of abuse. I discussed previously how repetition creates strong neural pathways. Even in adversity, those pathways strengthen. This means that our brain does not have to put more energy into trying to figure out what will happen next. Even if the outcome is dismal, we have an understanding that we have survived it in the past. So, when the trauma is consistently firing on the same neural pathways, the damage is not as great.

In contrast, if the trauma is unpredictable, the brain is constantly working overtime to build new pathways to try and make sense of what is going on in the environment. There is no strengthening of the myelin sheath. There is no understanding of having previously experienced the event and being confident of survival. So, the brain spends a lot more development trying to figure out ways to protect itself. The brain spends more energy making new dysfunctional pathways.

When we think of developing new neural networks and pathways, it is repetition that builds the myelin strength surrounding them. When my son was learning to ski, he became less fearful and his pain decreased the more times he fell. He knew he could get back up. He had a lot of practice not actually dying. In the morning, he was convinced he would die if he fell on the bunny hill. By the afternoon, he had fallen enough to disprove his rather convincing self-narrative. He pruned the weaker pathway of defeat and grew a strong pathway of success.

The more predictable and later in life our social/emotional/cognitive trauma (adverse experience) is, the better our outcome. This is because the foundational systems of our brainstem, limbic, and diencephelon are formed early. Physical trauma is the opposite. With the exception of trauma to the head, physical trauma has a much better outcome earlier in life. The reason is because the physical body is growing and thereby changing quickly in early life. Those of us over forty years of age are keenly aware of how much slower the physical body heals the older we get.

During infancy, our neurons are forming foundational pathways for attachment, heartbeat stabilization, temperature control, sleep, bowel and bladder function, and hunger/satiety patterns. Damage at this time is severe. If we have disruptions when the brain is learning to sleep, we lose that ability to self-soothe and relax. If you've ever been sleep deprived, you understand how much that state impedes functionality. Sleep deprivation can even lead to diagnosable acute psychosis. Adverse experience that occurs very early in development is really hard to overcome, because SO much depends on being able to sleep, eat, attach, and move your bowels. The timing and type of adverse experience matters a lot in regard to our neurobiology.

The hope I offer in these stories of childhood trauma is that we don't have to be perfect parents. Indeed, that isn't actually what is best for our children. Often, mistakes that are repaired have more lasting positive impact on brain development than mistakes that are never made. Children need experiences that involve being uncomfortable followed quickly by comfort being provided by a loving caregiver. We must be shown empathy to be empathetic. Our brains and sensory systems simply do not develop in isolation. We need the slight stress to spike the adrenaline that cues the brain for learning. We need caregivers to accurately assess how we are feeling and mirror that back to us in words, historical stories, and non-verbal body language.

When a child misses a critical window of development, we must go back and re-teach these things. When an OT engages in sensory play, we aren't just handing a child a can of shaving cream or a bucket of rice to "fix the tactile system." The occupational therapist is giving the child those missed experiences with reflection, words, and connection. We say things like, "Ooh, that's sticky. You don't seem to like that because you are wiping it off. That's a tall shaving cream tower. Look how that shaving cream makes my hand look white like yours. What happens if we add food coloring? What do your eyes tell you? Oh! Now it's blue!" For the child who is hesitant, we might start with a pencil dipped in the shaving cream and slowly build on that foundation to immerse the entire hand. For the child that goes a bit too alert with the shaving cream, we might add more texture like water beads or cornstarch to give them more tactile input. We might recognize and respect their level of adventure and play with shaving cream in a large tub with a swimsuit so they can fully immerse themselves as if they were a toddler playing in a mud puddle or with mashed potatoes. We begin in their window of tolerance then slowly open it wider as we patiently work WITH them.

We find ways to identify what they are seeking and provide socially appropriate replacement behaviors. I remember a student I worked with in the past who needed to feel the sensation of spitting. Simply telling him to not spit or giving him consequences was not helpful or effective. Instead, we gave him a soda can to spit into. In rural Indiana where chewing tobacco was common, this adjustment switched the behavior from offensive to socially normative. Eventually, he no longer spit.

I find this approach helpful with many sensory-based behaviors that caregivers try to extinguish. First ask, "What sensory benefit does this have for this child?" Then ask,

"Is there a way to modify, adapt, reframe, or redirect this behavior to not be offensive?"

In addition, I have developed a screening question that I ask only in my head: "Is this behavior likely to stop the person from getting a second date?" This question does more than make me giggle. It also helps me write useful client goals. When talking this process through with parents, I love the example of nose picking. If someone picked their nose, would I give them a second date? Maybe. Did they use a tissue? Did they do it in private? These might be simple things that I could easily address and not make it a big deal. But if a person were to pick MY nose, I would not give them a second date. That is something I definitely would have to make a therapeutic goal to extinguish.

What about a verbal tic? Shaking ("flapping") of the hands? I might choose not to address these things unless they were very intense. When looking at a behavior, I consider whether it can simply be ignored, whether it's a developmental stage that may resolve on its own, and whether it is a battle I am willing to fight. I also consider to what degree it impacts long-term functioning. If my therapeutic intervention does not improve a person's function, I'm betting there are other things I could work on.

Another point to consider is that just because I CAN help with a sensory behavior, doesn't mean I need to. If it's not socially a turn off, I might leave it be. After all, how boring would our world be if we didn't all have adorable little quirks and sensory preferences that allow us to playfully discuss our wonderful differences around a campfire or barbeque dinner?

We learn and develop within the context of a relationship. When I began studying trauma, I didn't fully see that. Now, I can't unsee it. We were literally created in a relationship. Ideally, the two people who conceived us had a healthy relationship at our very beginning. Sadly, for many children we serve, their relational foundation was challenged at their very conception. Whatever our beginnings, it is through the seeking of and engaging in positive relationships that we live our most fulfilled lives.

SECTION TWO

The Sensory Systems

CHAPTER 6

SENSORY PROCESSING

Sensory processing involves three steps.

1. A sensory stimulus must occur, and be **received.**

2. The sensory stimulus is **interpreted** as a threat or a thought. Is this something that will hurt me, and do I need to respond immediately? Or can I think about it before I respond? While thinking about it, WHAT do I think about it? Do I like it? Do I dislike it? Should this stimulus alert or calm me?

3. We react or **respond** to the original stimulus.

The label sensory processing disorder indicates that there is a misconnect somewhere within these steps. The dysfunction can happen in any of the steps: receiving, interpreting, or responding. Sometimes the system is over- or under-responsive and the child doesn't register the stimulus at all. Sometimes they overreact to it. Sometimes they do not have enough exposure to the stimulus to understand how to interpret it within the social context. Most times, if an OT has been called to consult or treat, the response does not match the social context.

One of the confusing things about sensory processing is that the systems can often be independent of one another. A child may have no difficulty with the sense of taste but have great difficulty with touch and sound. A child can be over-responsive in one sense and under-responsive in another. To a person new to sensory processing disorder, this can be very confusing.

As we begin to explore these systems, you will see how they can be separate as well as collective. I like to say that nothing happens in isolation. When you eat, you engage your sense of taste, smell, and touch. For a while with food aversions, it is helpful to have a good OT on the team who is skilled in activity analysis. What part of the particular rejected food is causing the problem? Is it the texture, temperature, or taste? Is it the oral-motor strength or dexterity required to swallow it without gagging or choking? A simple task of chewing a piece of meat has many components that each need to be carefully analyzed in order to figure out why it is rejected. When we look at sensory processing, we must understand how the separate systems work collectively to create the complexity of the human sensory experience.

My interest in the sensory system began when I met Judy McRoberts, OTR. Judy was a school OT who allowed me to shadow her for a semester my senior year during my high school cadet teacher enrollment. I figured working in special education would be an ideal career path for me. I've always loved my dad's knowledge of medicine. But I loved my mom's schedule as a middle school math and Spanish teacher. While I enjoyed the teaching aspect, it was Judy who introduced me to OT, the career that would become my passion.

Judy's day was full of variety. She did crafts, made splints, modified fine motor and oral motor tools, and led sensory groups. It was amazing. I remember one day she had me set up a sensory obstacle course. For fun, I attempted to complete it myself, then asked, "How did I do?" She simply said something to the effect of, "You did great. You'll be a great OT. Many people who lack sensory skills understand it better." Ummmmm...what? What the heck did THAT mean? I didn't even know what "sensory" was. I definitely didn't think I had a lack of ANY kind of skills.

That was a humbling wake-up call, but I quickly pushed it to the back of my mind. I wasn't really interested in sensory stuff. I wanted to cure cerebral palsy! Of course, I was a high school senior brand new to the field of OT. It wasn't until I was accepted to OT school that I realized that there is no cure for CP. I also realized that I was not designed to work in an acute hospital setting where children sometimes don't survive. I lost two patients during my acute care internship and quickly realized I was destined to be a school therapist.

I chose to work in a rural setting in Indiana because my boyfriend at the time was studying at the town college. It was the best job I've ever had in my twenty-five years of being an OT. We truly had a dream team of therapists and related service coworkers. We worked well together and shared a passion to help the children we served. Of those, I quickly realized we had a disproportionate number of children with autism spectrum disorder. My biggest diagnoses on my caseload were autism spectrum disorder and difficulty with handwriting.

Having studied mostly physical disabilities in school, I felt ill equipped to treat either. So, I studied. I researched, I read, and I asked questions. I developed a curriculum to help my teachers help their students write. I discovered I LOVED teaching continuing education. I wrote several courses, including one titled, "Calming Strategies for Autism." After all, that was what the teachers really needed. There was much debate on the cause, diagnosis, etc., but at the end of the day, teachers needed to know how to stop getting bitten, hit, pinched, and screamed at. The children needed to feel safe, valued, respected, and included.

I had a great understanding of how someone with autism feels. My friend and colleague, Ann O'Neill-Schlosser, once described me to a new staff member. She said, "This is Marti. She walks into a room full of kids with autism and they start flapping their hands and jumping, saying, 'She's one of us!'" At first, I wasn't sure how to take that. I figured it meant I knew my stuff and I really did have a knack and subconscious understanding of the world of autism. I thought I was just perceptive.

It wasn't until many years later that my husband and I rented Temple Grandin's movie, *Thinking in Pictures*. There was a scene where it was explained how Temple sees spoken words. It was like a Rolodex of images flipping through her mind. My husband simply stated, "That's fascinating."

I was like, "Wait, what? You don't think like that?!?!?" I then completed several online autism "tests" and quickly realized it might not have been a coincidence that I related so well to that movie. I don't have an autism diagnosis. But I do think in pictures, have difficulty processing sensory input (especially auditory and tactile), and have to work really hard to understand social situations. I try and use those superpowers for good. I try to use them to help others understand how it feels to have a body and mind that don't always perceive things the way those around me do. Something my husband says about me that I find funny is, "Marti doesn't just think outside the box. She looks around the room and says, 'Wait, what box?'"

Judy was right. Those of us with sensory deficit really do have an inside understanding of how the systems work. I've made it my life goal to help others view sensory processing a little differently, and to help them understand the "skill versus will" idea, that even when we have the will, we can't operate beyond our skill without support. I experienced this myself with my two-year-old on that beach trip many years ago. I intensely dislike sand. I love to rent a beach view condo where I can see, hear, and smell the ocean without having to touch the sand. I love scuba diving, but only offshore where sand can't stick to me. I would label myself tactilely defensive toward sand.

When my sweet little two-year-old toddled out to me as I was in the surf washing the sand off my feet, she face-planted. The waves were about to drown her. I was paralyzed. I knew I needed to pick her up and save her.

But…she was covered in sand. I'm proud to say I was able to compose myself enough to scoop her up by the time the second wave arrived. I'm glad I had a year of summer lifeguard skills that I didn't need to activate. But it was a close call. I share this story to illustrate skill versus will. Every maternal bone in my body wanted to grab my child instantly. I definitely had the will to save her from the first wave. But my skill was inaccessible at that moment. The fear of the tactile onslaught I was about to subject myself to put my arousal zone into the freeze category.

Thankfully, my husband rushing towards me and the fear in my daughter's little eyes helped distract me enough to do what needed to be done. Sometimes the children we work with pull themselves together the same way. They have underlying sensory challenges, but they are able to push through. But it's absolutely exhausting. We see this a lot in the schools. For children with auditory challenges, they push themselves through the entire school day but fall apart the moment they get home. They can pull it together until lunch and then they just don't have the energy to keep that fight/flight/freeze at bay any longer. These sensory-triggered outbursts have very little to do with the specific people nearby, or with lack of desire to follow social protocol, and much more to do with trying to protect a defensive sensory system.

One exciting thing about being connected to the NMT community is that it has opened doors for me to have conversations with other professionals working in trauma. It has allowed me to attend conferences where I present for a few hours and then sit in on other presentations. The more I learn about trauma, the more I realize that the sensory system holds a pretty big key to helping children who have experienced adversity. I connected the dots that the sensory system develops really early, is incredibly relationally impactful, and is in many cases a large puzzle piece for parents and non-OT caregivers as to the why behind many behaviors connected to trauma.

During a recent call with the Texas Juvenile Justice Department, we were discussing sensory strategies to help one of the teens in their system and I noticed that many of his documented aggressive behaviors involved his mouth. He yelled a lot, spit, bit, and tried to swallow non-food items. He seemed very orally focused to me. Gum isn't allowed because (news to me) gum can be used to "gum up" the locks to rooms and prove a safety risk. But I wondered if we could maybe offer frozen foods that would increase oral motor input. What about frozen licorice, frozen peas, or frozen Tootsie Rolls?

If his mouth was occupied with a proprioceptive treat, I hypothesized that it would be unavailable to hurl slang and bite flesh. Another child tended to do a lot of self-harm and after angry outbursts often had "no idea" why he was so angry. I see a child who isn't very in touch with his feelings and is seeking proprioceptive input to help him know where he is in relation to himself and others. Remember how we initially learn our sense of self through the eyes of others. Others see and describe our outsides. But many children did not get this loving introduction to who they are. If they don't understand the outer senses, the inside, or hidden, senses are even more unknown to them. The counselor and I discussed ways to increase physical activity and we brainstormed a few tactile fidgets that would be safe in the dorm such as sponges, washcloths, soft Koosh balls, shaving cream, pudding, and water beads. While I have no idea what cognitive strategies would be effective for these teens, I know if their mouth and proprioceptive system aren't calm, their actions will reflect that. I believe my job as the OT is to help the specialists calm the bodies so that they can treat the minds.

Over years of giving trauma-informed sensory talks, I have learned that attendees value the tips for calming versus alerting (discussed earlier in this book) as well as the breakdown of the individual senses. That breakdown will be the focus of the next chapter.

CHAPTER 7
THE HIDDEN SENSES

I'll start with the "hidden senses" of proprioception, the vestibular sense, and interoception. My friend Michael Remole, LCPC, brilliantly describes these senses as the wind in our sails. We don't necessarily see these senses or the things that affect them. But these are the senses that really drive the ship, or our body. If these senses are not functioning properly, our ship/body may move erratically from too much input or it may stall out without enough. When the wind is "just right," it sets the sails so that we can sail our course correctly. We have control of the rudder (reason and decision making) and we can meet the goals of our destinations.

PROPRIOCEPTION

The proprioceptive sense is how we know our position in space. It tells us how our joints and muscles are moving and how heavy or light an object is. It is the ability to walk down a hallway without touching the walls or pick up a full cup of water without spilling it. It is the ability to pet a bunny without squishing it or hug a person "just right."

The proprioceptive sense travels from the input site of the sensory receptors located in the muscle bellies, tendons, and bone joints up the spinal cord to the thalamus to the sensorimotor cortex. I sometimes describe these receptors visually as the little fluid-filled candy beads at the frozen yogurt shop. As the muscles contract and pull the bones to flex the joints, these little beads release the neurochemicals that travel up the spinal cord to tell the body where it is in space. The harder the joints contract, the more chemical is released. So, the more firm or intense the pressure, the more information is transmitted. There are a few anatomical loopholes here, but it provides a nice visual explanation.

When the proprioceptive sense is not correctly interpreted, a child may be very rough. They have difficulty knowing how much force they are using with their muscles. They may feel like they are being hit or shoved when someone simply bumps lightly into them. They may have difficulty walking down the hallway without touching every piece of artwork being displayed within arm's reach. They must touch EVERYTHING because they are relying on their tactile and visual sense to tell them where they are in relation to other objects. Often, when one sense is not providing adequate input, children will rely heavily on other senses to compensate. A simple way to screen for this compensation is to have the child close their eyes and ask them to demonstrate various body postures such as touching their nose or pointing to the ceiling.

Therapeutically, I believe the proprioceptive activities that simultaneously stimulate the deep touch receptors are the powerhouse intervention. My hypothesis for this lies in the anatomy and my clinical observations. Understanding the ways different sensations are received and transmitted has been vital to my work as an OT in settings from outpatient rehab to inpatient pain management. For others interested in learning more about neuroanatomy, I highly recommend Penn State neuro professor Dr. Marc Dingman's *2-Minute Neuroscience* series on YouTube.

Nerve tracts that carry touch and proprioceptive information enter the spinal cord at various levels. There are many different types of sensation-transmitting nerves that are bundled within the tracts. Touch receptors involved in light touch, pain, and temperature follow along the spinothalamic tract, which carries information about survival. Pain and temperature are easily viewed as immediate threats. Light touch needs a bit more context. In earlier times, wind changes meant weather changes. Humans needed to be sure they had appropriate shelter for the climate. Hair in the eyes obstructed the view of predators. Snakes, spiders, and poisonous plants brushing lightly against the body could lead to harm if undetected. Today, our bodies interpret light touch as a threat, even when our modern society has less true threat coming in from our light touch receptors.

Once the neurons carrying threatening sensations enter the somatosensory cortex, we develop an understanding of type and location of the stimulus. With pain, before the information reaches the cortex (thinking area) the withdrawal reflex is engaged to cause an immediate withdrawal from the pain. This withdrawal reflex is unconscious and happens quickly.

Stepping on a LEGO ultimately leads to thought. But that thought process happens after the withdrawal reflex. When the LEGO hurts our foot, the amygdala (a brain structure involved with memory) signals, "Remember this pain. Let's not step on those again. Pssst...Hey, Cortex, make the kids pick up those LEGOs in the future." But the **immediate** response of removing the painful stimuli happens quickly, reflexively, and unconsciously. This is an important concept as we work to develop compassion for the children we serve who have very quick, seemingly over-reactive responses to light touch and painful stimuli. When we can understand the anatomy involved for the child to receive and process the information, we can better understand why light kisses from a heavily perfumed aunt, or a classmate simply brushing against them can cause a true fight or flight response. They literally aren't able to **think** about how to respond to those types of sensory input before the reaction is made.

Proprioception follows primarily along the dorsal columns-medial lemniscus and the spinocerebellar tract. It is not perceived as a threat by the thalamus, so is sent to the cortex to be "thought about," before reaching the motor neurons. How hard is the item? How heavy is it? How much muscle power is needed to move this item? You

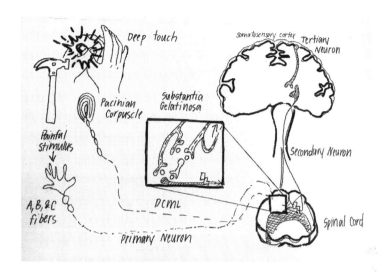

pick up a glass that is lighter than you thought it would be, and you spill your drink. You miss the last step that you anticipated and you stumble a few steps before your feet catch up. When we feel threat or danger, our brain goes into protection mode and we literally stop thinking. We engage reflexes that physically remove our body from harm's way and provide postural stability so we don't fall over. Due to its incredible anatomy, proprioceptive sensory information engages the cortex. It's a way into that thinking brain to start to process trauma and calm ourselves down.

Another significant anatomical concept is that proprioceptive activities **that involve deep touch** *override* the fight or flight response. Deep touch sensory receptors synapse in a part of the spine called the *substantia gelatinosa*. This structure is commonly called the "Gate" and plays an important part in a neurological theory called Gate Control

Theory. This theory explains how a neurotransmitter called *enkephalin* acts as a "gate" to block pain sensations from reaching the brain. **Deep touch stimulates chemicals that inhibit pain sensations**. This is why rubbing an injury immediately after the sensation registers helps it feel better. While proprioception is defined as knowing where our body is in space, **"proprioceptive activities" often include deep touch**. In order to push the joints together and flex the muscles in these proprioceptive activities, the skin is often pressed firmly and simultaneously. It amazes me that neurologists now have research that supports what loving caregivers have known for decades—a hug or rubbing someone's back really does block the pain from the brain.

When we look at this graphic, we can see that the deep touch and pressure nerve receptors are much deeper in the skin than the pain and temperature receptors. The

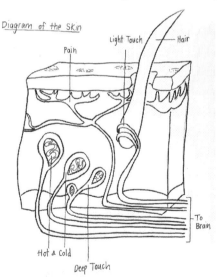

Diagram of the Skin

Light Touch — Hair

Pain

To Brain

Hot & Cold

Deep Touch

sensations that cause quick reactions are located closer to the surface of the skin and are therefore easier to stimulate, even accidentally. While temperature receptors appear to be deeper in the skin, temperature conduction is quick, and the stimulation can reach those receptors quickly. Heat transfers to cold, so a hot stimulus will likely register even faster than a cold stimulus since our skin temperature is closer to boiling than freezing.

To develop resilience, we need to have repeated sensory neural experiences of not being okay followed by a caregiver helping us feel okay. In infancy, there are hundreds of needs presented as little adverse experiences each day. When we consider how caregivers meet these needs, we discover that the infant received hundreds of caregiver responses activating the proprioceptive and deep touch senses. We press on the teething gums. We use firm pressure to secure a diaper. We pat their backs in a rhythmic fashion when they have gas. We swaddle and snuggle them close as we rock them to sleep. When a bee stings a person, they rub the area. We rub our head when we bump into a cabinet. We even press our lips into an open wound when a child lifts a cut finger to a caregiver. I cringe to think of all the germs being transmitted directly into the bloodstream from that kiss. But it is a very common connected, deep touch, nurturing response to a minor yet frequent childhood injury.

As we get older, we still rely heavily upon proprioceptive activities. As a member of a Motocross racing family, I saw many individuals that would probably fit the diagnosis criteria for hyperactivity disorders. But when they got on that bike, or in that car, they became calm and focused. If you've ever been to a dirt track, you probably can still feel deep in your proprioceptive memories the rumble of those engines and the buzz as they pass the stands. Michael Phelps is a well-known example of an athlete diagnosed with

ADHD who found swimming (a very resistive activity that puts pressure on the muscles and joints) to be very calming. Even when we have emotional pain, a hug within a trusted relationship brings calm. Jumping up and down when we are really excited helps keep us focused. When we are really angry, forcefully hitting something – or the classic toddler move of flopping forcefully to the ground – stimulates the cortex via the proprioceptive system and the deep touch pressure of our flopping limbs helps to calm. When we eat chewy, soft foods (I'm looking at you, breads and carbs), we engage the proprioceptive system. Walking, running, swimming, boxing, and many other things help stimulate that pain-override system. Many of these proprioceptive activities continue to be relationship driven, even into adulthood. **Proprioception is how we know where we are in relation to our social circle.** It's how we physically connect through hugging, fist bumps, etc. **Proprioceptive activities are how we *relate* to others.**

We can also view the proprioceptive system in the context of behaviors that aren't as socially acceptable. Binge eating, fighting, even aggressive sexual encounters can be viewed as ways to stimulate the proprioceptive system. When we look at these behaviors, we can see the common thread of attempts to pair proprioceptive activity with connection. As an OT who desires to understand the "why" behind sensory behavior, I find it important to look at these proprioceptive behaviors through a lens of connection and relationship. If a child from a hard place did not receive the rhythmic, repetitive, relationally rich patting, bouncing, feeding, and hugging, is it possible they are using these "deviant" behaviors to try and achieve that calm they are missing? How can we work together to replace these behaviors with other activities that will meet the need in a healthier way? My hope is this book (as well as the KALMAR app referenced at the end) will serve as a guide to help you do that.

Proprioception also works in tandem with many other senses. For example, music not only stimulates the auditory sense, but it's felt. Bright lights cause eyes to squint, providing proprioception through the eyelids, which prevent complete over-stimulation. Chewy foods are relaxing and taste yummy. When we jump, swing, slide, and spin, we feel gravity pull against our body to alert us and put pressure on our skin and joints to calm us. Proprioception pairs with more alerting stimuli to help maintain a "just right" level of arousal. Incorporating deep touch and proprioceptive activities throughout the day taps into our history of thousands of daily opportunities our caregivers used to help us feel safe and calm. Our limbic system remembers that we have felt this before, and it turned out okay.

Even a sharp inhale of a smell stimulates the muscles around the nose to contract and engage in the proprioceptive sense. Ever notice how you smell things that aren't pleasant in a quick, short burst but we pause and slowly inhale for pleasurable smells? That quick muscle contraction stimulates proprioceptors. This quick inhale facilitates the balancing calm for the incoming alerting smell. As I studied polyvagal theory and the parasympathetic (PNS) and sympathetic nervous system (SNS), I learned that during the inhalation phase of a breathing cycle, the SNS facilitates a brief acceleration of heart rate. During exhalation, the vagus nerve secretes a transmitter substance (ACh) which causes deceleration of the heart rate. As we look at muscular patterns and the joint movement while breathing, we can also see that the inhale breath causes the shoulders to move upward and extends the spinal column backwards. The exhale breath moves the body into flexion and midline posture. Anatomically, flexion pushes the joints together, squeezing on the proprioceptive receptors. Extension pulls the joints apart, decreasing the stimulus of the proprioceptive receptors. Because of this, it is recommended that the OUT breath be longer than the IN breath when using breathing techniques as an attempt to calm a person.

So how does childhood trauma affect the proprioceptive system? First, let's consider neglect. These children simply didn't get those repeated calming repairs. They did not get those thousands of rhythmic and repetitive experiences that built a neural framework for overcoming uncomfortable or painful things. With physical abuse, they were shoved too hard and never felt that attachment connection paired with the proprioceptive override. Some children even become head bangers or self-injurious as they try to provide this input to themselves in extreme ways. They cause physical pain in rhythmic, proprioceptive and deep touch ways to override their emotional pain. They haven't experienced that hugs, pats, humming, and going for a walk together are less harmful ways to get that input.

When we view proprioception as both the calming sense and the connecting sense, we can see how children who have difficulty with relationships tend to be over alert. They do not have those connected hugs, high fives, and hand squeezes to bring them back to calm. They may seek that proprioceptive input in other ways like the previously mentioned motorsports. They may crash into things with more pressure than is viewed as socially appropriate. They may be extreme risk takers. They may seek connection in overly physical ways such as aggression, yelling, and banging things around.

How do we help a child who demonstrates these "seeking" proprioceptive behaviors? Many OTs for years have created sensory obstacle courses. Indeed, The Karyn Purvis Institute of Child Development staff even used those in their early research camps. What I think many teachers, parents, and even some therapists miss in their sensory diets is the cognitive component. The connection between proprioceptive stimulation and cortical "awakening" is one reason we don't just have kids jump aimlessly on a trampoline. We also have them throw bean bags at letters, do math facts, sing songs, and answer questions. We engage the cortex while stimulating the arousal systems to help a child better move through the calm and alert continuum and begin to self-regulate. It is important that the caregiver be connected during these moments. Without a calm caregiver leading the activity, the child may become over alert and an opportunity for learning is missed. The cortical awakening is dependent upon guidance and connection.

We mirror the child's arousal level through rhythm with hand claps, music, and even our own bodies mirroring their movements. We gaze in the child's direction and give them verbal praise as they complete the tasks. When we therapists consider home programs and suggest that children carry over activities we engage in within our sensory gyms, we must remember they were **with us** in that gym. I've seen many home programs that suggest a trampoline or swing and the parent sends the child to the backyard alone to engage in the sensory input. But the child misses the relationship piece. They miss the mirroring of the regulated therapist who is using rhythm and repetition to influence the level of calm or alert during the sensory stimulation. Swinging in the backyard alone is very different from swinging in a therapy gym where the therapist is connecting with the

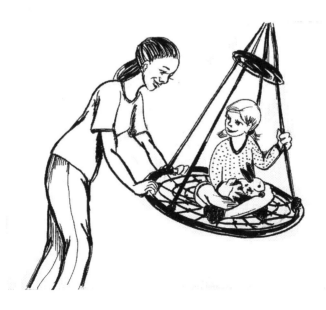

child via proprioceptive, cognitive, deep touch, or auditory input.

For those who have a more complex history with people, an idea I have found successful is to introduce non-people therapeutic tools like animals, weighted blankets, Lycra, heavy therapy mats, or stuffed animals. I once worked with a child who was selectively mute. She did not want to talk to me for our first session. While I completely respected this and certainly could understand some of her non-verbal communication, I wanted to know if she felt safe on my therapy swings. I wanted to help bring about that "just right" state, the state that alerts the child enough to make strong connections, but not so much that it puts them into fear.

Since she would not communicate with me, I wondered if she would respond to a litter of new baby bunnies at my home. It was amazing. She LOVED those soft fuzzy bunnies. I probably overstimulated their sweet little vestibular systems a bit, but she found her voice when I asked her to hold a bunny on the swing and let me know if they were scared or wanted more. She learned that when she provided "just right" deep touch and proprioceptive input to the rabbit, the rabbit got very still and calm. She was then open to consider what types of "just right" deep touch and proprioceptive input her mom could give her to help her be calm.

It was one of my very favorite therapy sessions of my entire career. I was so inspired, I called my farmer friend, Jamie Tanner, in hopes of creating more opportunities to use animals for building therapeutic relationships with children who have experienced adversity. A few short months later, the idea of Simple Sparrow care farm was born. Five years later, Jamie is writing a curriculum to share care farming with the world as she transforms so many lives within our small Texas community. You can learn more about her work at the end of this book and at www.SimpleSparrow.farm.

Weighted items that the child has complete control over, including stretchy materials like Lycra or Spandex, are very beneficial. Aside from providing compression to the joints and deep pressure over the skin, these items provide a sense of agency and control for the child. Children can grade the amount of pressure they provide to themselves and can control when and how the proprioceptive stimulation is provided. When a child feels they have lost control, they are desperate to get it back, to the point of destructive or relationship-damaging behavior. I encourage any relationship building opportunity for the child to regain that feeling of control.

I am often asked specifics about weighted items. When they first became commercially available in therapy catalogs, there were studies about how much weight was safe. These studies were mostly done with vests and backpacks. The findings were fairly consistent that a therapist should add no more than twenty percent of the child's body weight to a weighted vest (or backpack) and that the child would habituate (get used to the weight) after thirty minutes, at which time it was recommended to wait ninety minutes before re-applying it.

Newer studies using weighted blankets and other items find a high degree of variability in how much weight is preferred. It is also more difficult to arrive at conclusive guidelines given that the entirety of a weighted blanket would not be on the person at one time. A twenty-pound blanket may have two or three pounds on each side that is resting on the bed or chair, rather than on the person's body. In some blankets, the channels that hold the weight are far apart, allowing the weight to move around freely. This movement can be considered light touch and thereby counteracts the deep touch/proprioceptive intent of the blanket. I'll discuss more specifics about my favorite weighted product company, CapeAble®, in the tactile section.

When placing a weighted item on a person, it is important that they maintain a sense of control over it. I once provided a weighted vest for a child in a classroom who tended to wander aimlessly and was often trying to leave the building unattended. I returned to the classroom one day to a glowing review that the vest was working wonderfully. Then I noticed that someone in the classroom had doubled the weight in the pockets. The child wasn't moving around as much anymore because he physically did not have the muscle endurance to carry that weight. In this instance, this vest would be considered a restraint and would be illegal in most school districts. Therapeutic tools, and especially weighted or restrictive/stretchy items, must be easily and quickly removable.

I've been asked about using weighted blankets with people who have experienced sexual abuse. At first glance, this seems like a terrible idea, especially if the abuse involved being held down or restrained in some way. However, I have worked with residential facilities that leave weighted blankets out as free choice items, and I have heard reports that the blankets are well-tolerated and even provide a sense of protection. Consequently, I no longer hesitate to offer this tool to any population. I do, however, emphatically ensure that the user feels safe and in control at all times.

Lycra (or the brand name Spandex) is relatively inexpensive, lightweight, and can be graded by pressure depending on how tight you pull it. I love Lycra so much that I've been nicknamed "The Lycra Princess." (My friends initially proposed Lycra Queen. But the queen has way more responsibility. I prefer to be the princess.) The best kind of Lycra is one with a four-way stretch. It can be stretched uniformly across the body, thus applying even pressure on those one-and-a-half-inch to two-inch areas of nerve receptors. The more the person stretches the Lycra, the greater the input on the proprioceptive and deep touch receptors.

Another benefit of Lycra is that it usually pulls a person into the therapeutic position of flexion, in which the body comes towards midline. We naturally tend to go into this position when we are sad, by bending forward and flexing our head downward. Conversely, when we are excited and joyful, we extend our limbs out and lift our head upward. I observe these tendencies at play when someone is upset and we touch their back—this touch tends to alert them more, and they extend. But when we lower ourselves below their eye level or hug them forward, they tend to calm.

This is one reason I get so frustrated with takedown techniques that force a person onto their back. This position anatomically and neurologically escalates alert behavior. I recognize that pushing someone face forward into the floor has its own contraindications, so I haven't yet worked out a great solution. But I do think it is important to understand what happens biologically and why someone may take longer to calm in a takedown situation than we expect. Ultimately, it would be wonderful if we could understand escalation tendencies well enough to intervene earlier, preventing the need for a takedown in the first place. I sincerely hope that as we become more trauma informed, we will decrease the use of force in behavior interventions.

Deep touch massage can be a very intimate activity, and some of the individuals we treat may not find it comfortable. But we can offer other neurologically-informed strategies. A weighted blanket, therapeutic trigger-point tools, or even animal-assisted therapy can all be good alternatives. A child once explained to me how a snake wrapping around his arm felt like an arm hug. Not everyone likes the same sensations or specific ways to stimulate their senses. However, the biology of the senses tends to be universal. As we understand how human anatomy is designed to interpret and react to sensory stimulation, we can better understand what the person is seeking and find ways to replace the non-preferred activity with one that is more socially accepted.

It is important to remember that systemic change occurs when alerting/stress-inducing input is paired with relational, deep touch, cognitive override. To me, the three legs of the stool are relationship, proprioceptive activities involving deep touch, and target sensation. The target sensation is whatever sense we are pairing with deep touch and relationship in a therapeutic activity. For example, simply sending a child out to a swing set (the target sensation) as part of a "sensory diet" will likely just continue to alert them. However, if we go out with them, stand behind them, and push on their backs each time they swing toward us, we have added deep touch and relationship. You get similar benefits by having them jump off the swing and land in something soft as you cheer them on. Instead of just jumping erratically on a trampoline, have them jump to the cognitive rhythm of a song you sing in the context of relationship. Add a few seat drops here and there on the trampoline for a little extra proprioceptive input.

Proprioceptive Deep Touch = Relational Calm. As a general rule, when a person engages in proprioceptive input, the effects will last up to four hours. Therefore, when planning a sensory diet, it is best to incorporate intentional proprioceptive input four to five times per day.

Below is a list of deep touch/proprioceptive activities

SPORTS	FAMILY	DAILY ACTIVITIES
Martial Arts Gymnastics Ice Skating Skiing Tennis/Racquetball Golf Baseball/Cricket	Pillow Fights Hugs Trail Biking Hand Shake/Clap Routines Couch Cushion Burrito Couch Cuddles Couch Cushion Crash Pit Legos Hot Lava	Kneading dough Eating chewy foods/gum Rolling Dough/Cookies Mixing Food by hand Chopping Veggies Gardening/Raking leaves/shoveling Mowing the Lawn Brushing a pet Mechanical repair (hammers, vibration of saws)

HOBBIES	FRIENDS	SELF-CARE
Horse Back Riding Swing Dancing Line Dancing Stomp Dancing 4-Wheeling/Motor Sports Beatboxing/Rapping Large stroke painting (murals, rolling pins)	Walking/Jogging Group Drumming Swimming Parkour Ninja Warrior Courses Group Exercise Jumping on targets on a trampoline Hopscotch Tether Ball Cup Song routines	Massage Lotion on hands or feet Washing hair Wrapping up in a warm towel Body percussion (self-tapping)

with strong relational properties compiled with help from OTs from the Facebook group, Trauma Informed OTs.

Helpful Tips for the Child Who Crashes and Bumps Into Everything:

- Provide ways for the child to safely receive proprioceptive input. Jumping on cushions, crashing into pillows, jogging, swimming, and horseback riding can be great ways to gain this sensation.
- When able, add a relational component to the proprioception. Hug if it is safe and tolerated. If hugs are not perceived as safe, weighted blankets and Lycra sheets can provide similar stimulation. Do the proprioceptive activity side by side. Sharing a mirrored experience such as cuddling on the couch in separate blankets or walking side by side helps repair the developmental healing that many of these children missed early in their lives.
- Refer to the sensory diet and sensory room suggestions on page for more detailed examples on page 117.
- Firmly but not painfully rub textures on the body such as towels and washcloths to bring awareness to the tactile and proprioceptive systems.
- Pillow fights and "fake wrestling" in a safe and playful manner to stimulate the proprioceptive

sense with a strong relational component.

- Utilize clothing that adds compression such as Under Armour brand or a soft garment that is a little tight.
- Clothes with hoodies and pockets can be used to increase the pressure of the garment to a pleasing level of tightness.
- Cuddle with a large dog or fat cat to provide relational weight and snuggles. This can be a perceived safer option for individuals who have been hurt within

VESTIBULAR SYSTEM

Where deep touch paired with proprioceptive input is the powerhouse for relationship and calming, the vestibular system is the powerhouse for controlling regulation. It calms **and** alerts. Early in my journey to understand sensory processing, I took a course by Julia Harper, OTR/L. She referred to the vestibular system as "Mr. V," and described him as a Mafia boss, controlling the other senses in the background. If you have ever had vertigo or an inner ear infection, you may understand just how much the vestibular system controls. You may have felt nauseous or dizzy. Your sense of light and noise may have been muffled or amplified. When our senses become over-stimulated, it often makes us really irritable. We function best when things are predictable. When our body communicates something unexpected, we become fearful, and our brain moves into protection mode. This shift activates the limbic system and brainstem, and shuts down our frontal cortex, which leads to difficulty with reasoning and relationships.

Anatomically, it makes sense to compare the vestibular system to a Mafia boss. The vestibular system is in the middle part of the brain and begins to develop with the spinal cord. When the vestibular system is activated, often the eyes and spinal column activate along with it. This activation helps keep the body upright. Many of the primitive reflexes coordinate with the vestibular system to support gross motor physical development. For example, if you hold a baby upright, then tip her forward so her head faces the ground, her legs will begin to reflexively step, as a pre-walking exercise. If the head moves backward, she will reflexively extend the arms as if making the letter "y" to protect the head from impact.

When this development is hindered, reflexive movement can cause difficulty later, in school age children. Head movement contributes to activation of reflexes, and desk placement impacts head movement. When attempting to help a child focus, the teacher might put the "squirrely" child in the front of the class to keep them in arm's reach for tactile cueing. However, this then forces the child, who is already on a high alert state, to constantly be extending his neck as he looks at the teacher or board. Subconsciously, this child may flex his head and look down more to try and combat this posture. However, this is then seen by the teacher as disrespect and not paying attention. When the child is moved to the back of the room, they may surprise the teacher with better attention. An added bonus is that the child can see the entire room in their visual field without having to scan from side to side and engage the vestibular system.

The biggest job of the vestibular system is to protect the head from the pull of gravity and keep it upright and off the ground. Not only does this developmental Mafia boss develop early, receiving input as it floats around in the womb, but it also pairs with the cochlear (auditory) system. Cranial nerve VIII is the vestibulocochlear nerve, which innervates both auditory and vestibular nerve stimulation. If you have ever heard your favorite music jam and wanted to boogie, you have experienced this paired sensation. If the vestibular system is the Mafia boss, music can often calm his soul and become a powerful pairing stimulation. The auditory sense will be discussed more soon.

Notice the position of the vestibular nerves in this diagram:

The nerves connect to the semicircular canals within the

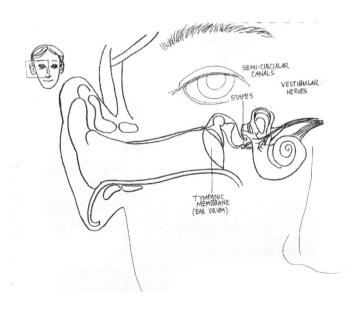

inner ear anatomy. These canals also contain fluid and hair-like projections called cilia.

The fluid and the cilia move in response to a change in our head position, and that information is conveyed to the brain by the vestibular nerve, to help us understand where our head is in relation to the floor. When we have an ear infection, this fluid doesn't move freely and therefore it is also difficult for the cilia to move freely and provide appropriate input. It is worth noting that when children are left in a crib to drink from a bottle often, when their environment is filled with smoke, or when they do not have adequate nutrition, the comorbidity of ear infections is great. If the developing system can't receive good data or input, it can't mature optimally.

Notice the three semicircular canals that are oriented in three different planes. Each canal detects a different movement. These movements are nodding up and down (like a "yes"), tilting left to right (ear to shoulder), and shaking side to side (like a "no"). The fluid and cilia move differently in each canal, based upon which way the head is moving. Getting information from each canal results in the most accuracy, and best supports us in keeping the brain safe within the skull, and off the floor. Two other structures also detect movement — the utricle (horizontal movements) and the saccule (vertical movements). Together, these structures detect motion, head position, and spatial orientation.

Because information from the vestibular sense is prioritized by the brain from the earliest days of development, it impacts our arousal level. If our head moves from top to

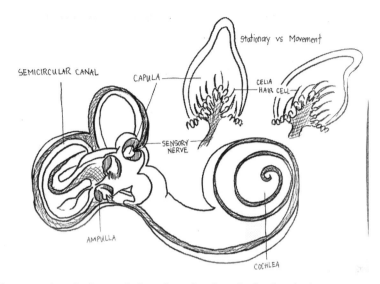

bottom (cephalocaudal, or head to butt), the brain interprets that as the most calming stimulation. Watch a caregiver do the "baby bounce" where they hold the baby against their chest and gently bounce up and down from their knees. Consider how many of these connected interactions an infant receives on a daily basis, and how effective they are in calming a baby. Patting the infant's back after feeding sends both proprioceptive and vestibular input up the spinal cord for a double dose of calming input. These connections are first formed in infancy through repetition with that connected caregiver. Without these repeated experiences, the infant who experiences early childhood trauma does not develop these neural connections in this healthy way.

While the up and down movement is most calming, front to back movement is the next most calming. If you have seen the movie *Rain Man*, you might remember how Dustin Hoffman swayed front to back when his character became upset. Moving forward and back in a swing or rocking chairs tend to calm the vestibular system.

After up-and-down movement and front-to-back movement, let's consider side-to-side movement, which tends to be perceived as neutral. Imagine a caregiver cradling an infant next to a crib, late at night. As the caregiver sways side to side, the infant receives the most calming cephalocaudal (head to butt) movement while the caregiver receives a more neutral side to side. The caregiver doesn't want to fall asleep **with** the infant; that would be incredibly dangerous. But they also don't want to wake up so much that they can't get back to sleep themselves. We can also observe this side-to-side movement in people waiting in line. They use neutral side-to-side movement to calm down a bit, but not so much that they are too calm to advance their place in line.

Elliptical movement can increase our arousal level. Consider a merry-go-round or a swing that is moving in wide circles, but not in a tight spin. Therapeutically, elliptical movement is often seen as the intermediate movement as we work to bring a child from overly alert into calm. It is important to note that there is also a rhythm about the vestibular sense. Since the input is graded along a continuum of arousal levels, the rhythm must be met in the context of relationship before the child can move between these levels. For example, it would be unsuccessful to expect a child to go from spinning around the room to sitting in a rocking chair. There must be transitional moves worked into the therapeutic interaction. When a child comes into my clinic very over-aroused and spinning, darting around, etc., I usually start them in a tight spin, like the twisted rope of a swing. The head of the child is moving in a clockwise or counterclockwise movement. Then I will use a transitional elliptical movement, where the head is continually facing one direction as the body moves through an oval pattern. Finally, I bring them into a rocking motion side to side, and then front to back.

This movement progression is gradual. If I move through the movement phases too fast, I lose the relational aspect and fail to match the energy of the child. We like to have our emotions and movement rhythm/rate mirrored to us. We want others to match us when we are in an alert state of arousal. If I move through these phases too fast or don't meet them in a high-alert state in the beginning, the child may not feel seen or validated.

Children who have built repetitive and strong neural pathways of being vigilant — perhaps to monitor the arousal level of an abusive caregiver — can pick up on this non-verbal communication with even more sensitivity. They have a lot of practice and neural firing to become over alert and therefore can have a strong desire to stay in a high arousal state by utilizing the vestibular system. So, when you observe a child spinning and you want them to calm, it is important to add some playful proprioceptive and deep touch input and help them work their way backwards within that vestibular continuum. Children with strong neural pathways of hypervigilance need repetition of new relational and deep touch experiences in order to form new neural pathways for calm. They need to learn that calm can be safe, and that they don't have to maintain a high alert status to achieve safety.

The tight spin is the most alerting movement to the vestibular system. Whenever I see a child engaging in a tight spin, I can guess that child is in a very alert state. Sometimes, they are in an overly alert state and the body has begun to dissociate. Thus, the child continues to spin without seeming to register any input. Some children who have built strong neural pathways to be alert and vigilant have a difficult time coming down into the calm state and will rely heavily on this spinning movement in their seemingly constant quest for more vestibular input.

The eyes and vestibular system are keenly connected. The eye muscles can even influence the vagus nerve stimulation of the stomach. (You get less motion sickness when the eyes fix on a faraway target.) Dancers and ice skaters rely on visual "spotting" to help regulate the vestibular system. When their eyes fix on an object, they are better able to monitor the input to the vestibular system and make slight adjustments to their balance.

The Post Rotary Nystagmus (PRN) test identifies how the body is regulating vestibular input, by observing how the eye muscles contract and relax rapidly, causing the eyes to move side to side or up and down, in response to vestibular input. I'll have the child who's in an overly alert state sit in an office chair, and I spin them at a rate of one rotation every one and a half to two seconds. When they stop, I will sit in front of them and have them look over my shoulder without focusing on anything. If the child is unable to "not focus," I ask them to simply close their eyes while I watch for the side-to-side movement of the eyes beneath their eyelids (understanding that closing the eyes can decrease how long the nystagmus lasts). Although there are different normative amounts based on the type of movement and age of the person, eight seconds is a good baseline for normal PRN in children. If you've never seen a post-rotary nystagmus or are curious to know what it looks like, find the child at the playground who is stumbling, and look at their eyes. It is almost certain they will be bouncing back and forth as the muscles contract and relax.

When nystagmus lasts more than eight seconds, I begin to wonder if the vestibular system is over-reactive. Oftentimes, children with over-reactive systems get car sick. They have difficulty with swings, they lose their balance often, and they tend to have more difficulty with interoception (which we will discuss next). When nystagmus is less than four seconds or non-existent, the system may be under-reactive. These children tend to be the daredevils. They can stimulate the vestibular system excessively and seem to never get dizzy. For these children, I have had success with changing the head position while I swing them. Often, I will use a platform swing or cradle them in my arms if they are small enough. When I spin them around while their ears are facing the ceiling and the floor, it engages a different semicircular canal. Most children are not skilled enough to do repetitive flips on a trampoline. Positioning the child in side-lying can stimulate those canals more efficiently. At the same time, they can stimulate the child's deep pressure sense with a weighted blanket or by rhythmically tapping the swing so that the child can feel it. I've seen increased PRN within only a few days when parents engage in this movement three times a day. This increased PRN indicates that the vestibular system is better registering the sensations.

When we consider the vestibular system through the lens of trauma, we must remember that the early experiences with caregivers provide neurological foundations. Even in the womb, maternal movement and the mother's sense of felt safety influence the development of this system. Studies show that early maternal stress is passed on to the developing baby as early as the first trimester, when the vestibular system is in the critical window of development. As the mother bends, reaches, and changes direction, those movements are passed through to the baby and influence this system's development. Movement that is patterned and predictable is easy for the vestibular system to interpret and respond to. A mother who walks, jogs, swims, rides a horse, or does other healthy lifestyle activities optimally stimulates the vestibular system. If the mother feels threatened and has a lot of sporadic movement paired with increased stress hormones early on, the baby develops with that irregular input. Domestic abuse can result in chaotic, arrhythmic input to the baby, as well as excess stress hormones that cross the placenta, all of which are detrimental to vestibular development. A mother who is high, depressed, or bedridden for medical complications is likely to be less active, which provides less than optimal stimulation to the developing vestibular system.

When using vestibular input in a sensory diet, consider that the effects can last up to six hours. Therefore, this input doesn't have to be offered as often. For a child with an under-reactive system (constantly seeking, low PRN), it is important to give them a "tight spin" opportunity or to combine the various types of movement in order to flood the semicircular canals with input, increasing opportunities for the child to register it. The brain can then retain the effect of that movement for much of the day.

INTEROCEPTION

The last of the "hidden" senses for this chapter is *interoception*. Interoception is the ability to perceive and interpret internal feelings, such as exertion, thirst, or anxiety. For this section, I reached out to my colleague, Kelly Mahler, OTD, OTR/L, who is an expert in interoception. She explained to me how there are two types of interoception — *implicit* (pulls information from things we don't consciously consider such as hormones, blood sugar, and blood pressure) and *explicit* (pulls information that has more conscious information such as hunger, cold, and safety). When we aren't proficient with our interoception interpretation, we may not feel our heartbeat or full stomach. But our body will give us additional clues such as hearing the thump in our chest or feeling the rhythmic vibrations against our ribs. Our skin (or clothing) gets tight when our stomach is stretched. These interoceptive organs function in a way that also engages other systems with more direct sensation

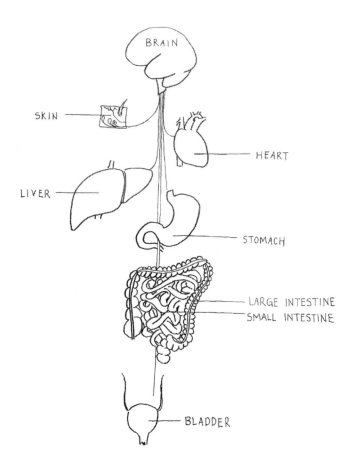

interpretation. As we expand our understanding of the many organs connected through the vagus nerve, we start to understand how to interpret patterns of the sensations we do feel. We start to see patterns tied with cognition and thought. When our skin sweats, our intestines rumble, and our heart races, we start to recognize that these feelings are associated with being nervous. Understanding the way our organs are connected helps us understand our internal feelings. Kelly states, "Being able to notice and interpret interoceptive body signals serves as the foundation of our emotional experience and is the very start of self-regulation. You need to understand how you feel in order to meet your needs successfully."

Studying trauma through the NMT and TBRI lenses reinforced ideas learned through my OT education, specifically how the brain and body are intimately connected. Occupational therapy was created during the first world war, when the human need for purposeful activity and emotional well-being was first being researched. OTs have been connecting the physical to the mental since the birth of our discipline. I am always excited to meet others who want to learn about our holistic profession. I can sum it up in a simple equation:

anatomy+psychology=occupational therapy

"If you can name it, then you can tame it." The challenge with interoception is that people often have a difficult time naming (or even noticing) how they feel, whether mentally, physically, or both. One of my favorite family inside jokes relates to something my daughter brought to our vocabulary when she was a toddler. It is the simple word, "Else." She requested a prolonged bedtime ritual: "I want a hug. I want Bunny to get a hug. I want water. I want another story. I want the night light on." Once she had exhausted all the requests she could identify as reasonable, she sweetly requested, "I want….else." It was a delightful use of language and if ever my husband or I are in a snacky mood where we probably should just drink water or find a healthy option, we simply say to each other, "I want….else." (When I say this, he usually brings me ice cream or popcorn. It's likely the "else" I wanted, but probably not the one I needed.) I find it to be a great way to describe to others the feeling of not knowing what else we want, need, or feel.

Dr. Perry's concept of state dependent functioning is all about who is driving the brain bus. When Limbic Larry is at the wheel, he's looking for fast food, immediate reward and safety. He is likely tired, stressed, or feeling big feelings. He doesn't have a lot of adjectives to describe the type of food he wants. As Cortex Charlie comes forward at the wheel for his shift, he has better access to those interoceptive cues such as blood sugar, thirst, and remembering what has already been ingested. He is relaxed. He has the capacity to look at a map and find the healthy farmer's market to buy better food choices. When our brain is in the back fight-or-flight zone, we rely on those patterned, repetitive, deep cow paths to know what "else" means until that frontal thought and reasoning area can be accessed to give us new skills and new pathways. When a child is wanting "else," it is a cue for the caregiver that they are functioning in the automatic zone of the brain. It is our cue that they are more likely functioning on skill versus will.

"Else" is the heart of poor interoception. We know our stomach needs "else," but we don't quite know what it is. Do we need to eat? Drink? Relax? Poop? Some children can't identify when they are thirsty or hungry or need to move their bowels. They may become constipated or dehydrated. They may over- or under-consume calories recommended for their size. They may have trouble knowing when they are fatigued and need to take a break.

When a child has poor interoception, they may have overwhelming or unclear information as to their current level of arousal. Without this awareness, they are unable to know how to relax their bodies to rest. They may have difficulty staying asleep. They may not ever feel tired. Not sleeping is a big deal. Sleep is when the body restores and heals, and lack of sleep can make an individual physically sick. It can make them groggy, short-tempered, forgetful, irritable, clumsy, and disconnected. Without restorative sleep, many well-intended therapeutic approaches simply won't be effective. Sleep is often one of the first goals I address with my own clients.

When we consider sleep through a trauma lens, we imagine how bedtime might have gone for that child. Maybe they didn't have a good bedtime routine. Maybe the home environment was chaotic and that is how the child developed their sleep habits. Once secure in a quiet, "safe" foster home, they may crave that chaos they came from. We can help by offering the level of noise they are used to along with some rhythm, repetition, and predictability. Maybe a white noise machine would be beneficial as the child learns to transition from extreme chaos to the safety of the new home.

Trauma impacts daily routines. Some children do not grow up with the warm bath and bedtime story. They lack the ritual and routine that begins to signal the brain for dissociation and falling asleep. For some, nighttime is associated with abuse, and the dark can signify imminent danger. Oftentimes abandonment occurs at night. Some children may be fearful of going to sleep because they don't trust that the caregiver will remain available through the night.

Unfamiliarity is another thing to consider. I travel a lot for conferences. I've noticed that I seldom sleep well the first night in a hotel. If I'm able to stay a second night, I always sleep much better. Recognizing this increased my empathy for children who are frequently moved within the foster system or with caregivers who are homeless or move frequently. They may have a constant thread of "first nights" that prohibit them from feeling safe and comfortable.

Getting good sleep isn't always as simple as creating a loving little bedtime routine and a soft blankie. Physical safety doesn't always equate to felt safety. For children who have experienced adversity, their safety rests upon their own shoulders. When they attempt to sleep, their safety feels threatened. They are fearful that when they close their eyes, something bad might happen. Until these children **feel** like they are safe enough to relax, sleep and rest will be very difficult to achieve. Children who do not feel safe need reassurance and repeated experiences that sleep doesn't have to be scary. A flashlight or a walkie talkie can provide safety by allowing the child to see in the dark or call out to a caregiver if needed.

In many families I work with, the parents are as exhausted as the child. When the child doesn't go to bed or fall asleep easily, the parent becomes frustrated, which is understandable. But this response can then reinforce to the child that bedtime is a time of parental disconnection. When I observe this situation, I often collaborate with the caregiver to find ways that they can be more rested themselves at bedtime. Can the caregiver set aside other evening commitments for a few weeks to establish a good sleep pattern for themselves? Maybe the dishes or laundry can wait until the next day or the weekend. Maybe bedtime can start earlier so that there is a time buffer for the child to ask for another story, a drink of water, or an extra hug. Sometimes these little moments of connection can help a child move from fear-based self-reliance to a more restful sense of security.

Tips for Better Sleep

- Co-sleeping in a room with an animal. Even a fish can provide a sense of not being alone or abandoned.
- Predictable sleep routines with lots of connection. Have intentional moments of alerting stimulation together paired with rich proprioceptive connection.
- Weighted or Lycra blankets to add proprioceptive input.
- A spray bottle of water to calm the imagination, with a "Monster Spray" or "Good Dream Spritz" label added. Adding a scent to the spray can be helpful. "If you smell like vanilla, you'll have sweet

dreams."

- Assuring the child that there is a grown-up home to keep them safe. Some children had to care for younger siblings at night, and they may need to be reminded that an adult is in charge at your house.
- Allow the child to sleep with a caregiver's T-shirt or other item of clothing to help them know they aren't abandoned.
- Allow the child to sleep on a pallet where they feel comfortable and secure, like in a caregiver's or sibling's room.
- Consider joint compression exercises or massage combined with low vestibular input, such as sitting in a rocking chair or swaying side to side to a lullaby, as part of the bedtime routine.
- Warm baths and uplifting stories as part of the bedtime routine.
- Night lights on timers so they help the child fall asleep, then turn off once the child is asleep. Motion sensor lights can be helpful for nighttime waking. Positioning is important so they aren't turned on if the child simply rolls over.
- Scented stuffed animals.
- A tent over the top of the bed to block out noise and/or light.
- White noise.
- Sleep music ("Weightless" by Marconi Union).

A child with poor interoception might perceive fear as

anger and lash out when he might be better served to seek safety. A child with poor interoception may not know how loud she is talking or might not be able to tell if she feels hot or cold. Interoception isn't just how we feel physically. It helps us know when we are emotionally distracted, anxious, or feeling joy as well.

Interoception can also be described as that wind in our sails. Even if our boat is in ship shape and seaworthy, if we have poor interoception, we will have no wind in the sails to guide the ship. Early childhood trauma greatly impacts interoception. In a healthy early relationship, the caregiver is repeatedly providing language (both verbal and nonverbal) while seeing the child's needs and meeting them. As needs are being met, the caregiver is giving description for sensations, emotions, and bodily functions. "Did you make a poo poo?" "Oh, that's so sad that your binky fell." "Good Nummy Nummy in your tummy." "Ooh, you are mad." "You are so tired. Let me rock you to sleep." So much of our first three years of life is someone helping us perceive how we feel and what we do and don't like, based on our body language and our relationship with them.

For some children, these conversations never happened. Some were left alone with no explanation for when/where/ how much they were supposed to eat. Other children's feelings were not merely invalidated; they were shamed. The caregivers may not have had the interoceptive awareness themselves to help a child learn to appropriately identify these sensations. Or maybe the caregiver was uncomfortable with negative emotions like fear and disappointment often associated with normal development.

We learn through patterned, predictable, controlled adversity. When our caregiver can't buffer this adversity for us and it becomes unpredictable and uncontrolled, we simply don't learn optimally. When the only emotions modeled for us are anger and disgust, we internalize those and don't know how to express fear and disappointment in ways that don't cause our bodies physical distress. When our caregivers send the message that they can barely handle their own emotions, we don't trust them with ours. So, we don't show ours. When we don't show our emotions to our caregivers, they can't help us "name them to tame them."

Although much of the developmental framework for interoception occurs during the critical window of birth to five, there is another critical window that opens up during adolescence and puberty. As the frontal lobe begins to mature, another round of emotional swinging and relational buffered discussion and identification occurs. So, while early intervention is best, later intervention can still be helpful.

The best way to help with interoception is to help the child notice how their body feels during playful engagement. Following the NMT model, we go back developmentally. With the infant, we first named external feelings—that's cold, smooshy, bumpy, soft, etc. As children get older, cooking can be a great way to discuss feelings and how they connect to our body. We make cookies. We talk about the sensation of each ingredient. How do they feel? How do they smell? How do they taste? Do we like the feel, smell, and taste? Is your perception different from mine? Can we compare the ingredients separately then combined? How do the tools feel? Can we engage the limbic system a bit and discuss memories surrounding food? Emotions? Are there certain foods that are comforting? Once we name the physical feelings, we can begin to name the internal feelings. Does this make you happy? Do you feel joy? Love? What about disappointment if the recipe burned?

What other activities can you think of? Swimming, horseback riding, and many other sports have sensory components and feelings that can be discussed. Arts and crafts, especially photograph-based collages, can be helpful. Sometimes it is difficult to identify our own feelings, but we can use cues from photographs and the distance of speaking about a third person to explore our own interoception. At Simple Sparrow farm, we often work with people to help identify an animal's suspected feelings before a child is ready to identify and discuss their own. Kelly has some great resources on her website, https://www.kelly-mahler.com, for those who are interested in practical, user-friendly ways to improve interoception.

I have found therapeutically that working on various movements can be helpful to bring awareness to internal sensations. By adding sensory information from the skin and proprioceptive receptors, we gain more information to understand how our lungs, heart, and other internal organs are functioning. Some movements are designed to physically manipulate internal organs. Stretching and stimulating the stomach in a clockwise direction as you face a person can help move things through the large intestines. Raising your arms up like you are making a standing snow angel can help with lung expansion. Something I notice in regard to lung support is that if a child does not have good core muscle tone in their abdomen and back, they will collapse forward and thus compress their lung capacity. The exhale is the calming breath while the inhale is the alerting breath. If a client can use their shoulders to lift up and get the air in, but they are too compressed to get the air out, they will be in a more alert state simply because of their breathing capacity in relation to their core stability.

As an OT, I'm often asking myself what sensory input a child is getting too little or too much of. Can I modify the environment to help them? Can I strengthen their system to better equip them for this input? Can I help them understand their internal cues? I work with the child either by exaggerating the input to make it easy to identify, or simply giving descriptive language repeatedly so that they may better express their needs.

In my years of providing therapy, I have found that when a challenge is visible, it is easier to give compassion. As a society, we are sometimes more compassionate with physical limitations. We widen the hallway or simply ignore when someone in a wheelchair makes marks down a thin hallway, but we become irritated when a child with an immature proprioceptive system must run his finger down the wall to understand his location. Understanding these hidden sensory systems inspires more compassion for the children we work with as they work so hard to rehabilitate these unseen differences. Understanding these hidden senses helps us raise flags to help see the hidden winds in the sails of children who experienced adversity.

MARTI SMITH, OTR/L

CHAPTER 8

THE KINDERGARTEN SENSES

When I was in kindergarten so long ago, the five senses of taste, smell, touch, hearing, and sight were all that were discussed. These senses tend to be more straightforward than our hidden senses covered in the previous chapter. In this chapter, I will explore how adverse experiences and early childhood trauma change the development and functionality of these kindergarten senses.

GUSTATORY: THE SENSE OF TASTE

Water is the sustainability of life. But food is quality of life. Taste is one of our first senses to come alive. We are born with a rush of tactile input. But the first real calming thing we do is eat. And we eat frequently. Infants are dependent upon the caregiver for their food. Touch can happen independent of other people. As a baby moves, the tactile system can be stimulated by things such as their clothing, furniture, pets, toys, even their own fingers. But food is 100 percent relationship-dependent from birth to several months of age. Even when babies are able to independently put the food in their mouths, they remain caregiver dependent for several years until they are able to independently meet their nutrition needs.

Food is a basic need, like clothing and shelter. When we are denied food due to neglect, poverty, or abuse, we are literally denied life. When we receive food, we receive care. Food is relationship. It fosters community. It celebrates our heritage and traditions. When I speak, I often ask attendees to try and come up with a cultural or community celebration that does not involve food. It is difficult to do. In times of distress, we often create meal calendars to help meet the basic need for food for the person who is hurting. We show them love through food.

I was considered a "feeding expert." Yet, my own child had feeding issues caused by a traumatic birth, my low milk supply, and my pride which caused me to resist simply switching to formula from the beginning. I wasn't in tune with my daughter's hunger cues, and she wouldn't accept the precious milk I worked so hard to pump. Even our positioning and her oral motor skills were impacted by my anxiety. I was force-feeding her with hundreds of different bottles trying to fix the "latch," but what I really needed to do was step back and focus on the connection.

This pattern continued into her toddler years, when I would make horrific green/organic/natural concoctions and insist that she eat them. We tried every diet known to the toddler interwebs. At one point, I actually stuffed ground chicken into gelatin capsules. The child was great at taking pills, so I tried to get protein in her that way. I only did it once. While creative and successful, I was able to see that "chicken pills" were an unsustainable level of ridiculousness.

It wasn't until her double digits that I let go a bit and allowed her to live off of potatoes for a year. (She ate a few other items, but potatoes were a consistent "yes" food.) People would ask if she was a vegetarian and we would lovingly reply, "No. She's a potatotarian." I received counsel from a dietitian friend that most picky eaters will expand their palate around the age of twelve. I held onto that with every believing bone in my body. Thankfully, my friend was correct. Our daughter did live on the potatoes-and-bananas diet for about a year. But over time, she increased her interest in cooking and baking, and her food choices started to expand.

She still won't eat meat or other complex textures. But she loves (and makes) a great soup, and her physical development is fine. She will also eat beans and an occasional egg breakfast taco. She is, after all, a seventh generation Texan and born Austinite. Her heritage would be in question if she always refused the iconic breakfast taco.

If I could offer advice from an expert who had her thoughts radically changed by experience, it would be this: People have survived on bananas. People have survived on grains. Our long-ago ancestors had very limited food choices and they survived. With deeper knowledge of brain development, I now understand the interplay between relationship and feeding. Granted, it took trying chicken pills! But I learned to shift the focus of feeding from content (six grams of protein in an egg; two grams of fiber in a taco shell) to connection (our shared heritage as breakfast taco people).

I believe that if you have the relationship, the food will follow. One of my friends ate her first salad while on a date with her now husband. Impressing him gave her the motivation to try a new food she had previously adamantly refused. But children who were neglected did not have relationship. They missed the pairing of hunger sensations with a loving caregiver telling them they are precious as their bellies filled. My own child's hunger was met by a caregiver consumed by shame and anxiety. Feeding was such a struggle that her belly often didn't fill completely. We repeated this non-connected scene many times each day. Without those positive feeding experiences, children are left to pair hunger with loneliness and isolation. Those little runner neurons make repeated pathways that become very deep lawnmower trails that either lead them to hoard food or reject it once it is offered by a new loving caregiver.

The very foundation of connection and human relationship begins with food. For children who have experienced adversity, food is a struggle. For some of them, there was a lack of exposure to food. For others, food was used to gain control of them. For many, there are deep rooted issues surrounding the gustatory sense.

Like many aspects of development, our oral motor skills develop in a sequence. Even the anatomy of the feeding chain changes as the child grows. At birth, the airway is anatomically designed for easier swallowing and breathing while drinking. The tongue moves forward and backward in a suckling pattern. Dexterity, or moving the tongue up and down and from cheek to cheek, doesn't develop until later. Without solid foods, there is little need to clear food from the non-existent teeth.

Everything from tooth eruption from the gums to tongue muscle development happens within a predictable sequence when children are exposed to food progression initiated by a loving caregiver. While suck/swallow/ breathe is one of the very first things to develop, many things can impact this progression. The lips of children born with medical complications such as a cleft palate may not form a tight seal, which prevents air from entering the mouth and allows food to go down the esophagus easily. Babies born prematurely are given nutrition via a tube down their throat. Therefore, they miss those hundreds of practice opportunities for neural synapse formation to begin to smoothly and automatically swallow without having to "think" about it.

When food is withheld from a child, they do not get these relational repetitions that help mature the neural networks. If you have ever seen a very hungry person, they can attempt to eat very rapidly. The suck/swallow/breathe sequence is off in rhythm and timing. If you've ever had your swallow timing interrupted, you may have experienced food going "down the wrong pipe." This is one reason children can appear to be very hungry one minute and then reject food the next.

Keeping our airway clear is a primitive response. There are many emotional triggers within the amygdala that are hard wired to keep our airways clear. Strong choking equals strong memory and food avoidance. I've heard many people who got sick after eating a certain food and, no matter how much they loved that food, they are unable to eat it again for a very long time. The body builds strong emotional memories to protect itself from re-traumatizing events that threaten our airways.

In addition to food triggers, children can resist food based on texture. To understand this better, we need to consider how our oral cavity develops. We begin with a thick liquid. Colostrum is thick. Milk has a thick texture. We don't give infants water because not only does it lack caloric density during the time in development where every calorie counts for future cell growth, it has a low viscosity, or is very thin in consistency. From thick liquids, we move to thick solids, such as rice cereal or purees.

There is a term in oral motor therapy called a *bolus*. This is a term that describes how easily a food clumps together as a compact mass in the mouth. As it sticks together, it goes down the esophagus in one piece that is easier to manage. Beginning foods are usually very thick and sticky, but also wet and slippery, such as bananas, avocados, and rice cereal. This makes them very easily form into a bolus and quickly go down the esophagus so the suck/swallow/breathe rhythm is smooth without requiring the still-developing tongue to do much of the work. Foods like steak or carrots would be choking hazards for infants, who have not yet developed the tongue strength and dexterity to manipulate those foods into a bolus.

Worth mentioning is the connection between feeding and language. Without the constant babbling and "mama," "lala," and "dada," the tongue may not develop sequentially. Therefore a child who does not get verbal stimulation could ultimately not develop tongue skills to eat some of the more nutritious foods later in life. Without the repetition of the lip closure with the relational "mmmmm" mirrored with the caregiver, the baby's lip muscles don't get as much muscle stimulation to strengthen for the more complex foods. This is just another example of how food is so inherently connected to communication.

When we break down how food consumption develops sequentially, it is easier to see where children from adverse experiences may have missed some of these foundational experiences. As they move forward, they may have poor oral motor skills that not only affect their speech, but also their nutrition. Many of the children I work with prefer starchy white foods. Rice, bananas, heavily processed chicken nuggets, pizza, cheese, potatoes, and goldfish crackers. While these foods appear to have different textures, they are all similar in the way that they form a bolus. Once they become wet with saliva, they clump together easily and slide down the esophagus without much skilled tongue movement or risk of choking. These also tend to be highly processed foods without dense nutritional content. The more nutritious foods such as carrots, beans, salads, and beef all require more tongue dexterity, strength, endurance, and coordination.

Once we see how the acceptance of nutritious food requires repetition of positive experience along with predictable developmental sequences, it is easier to understand how food can be such a complicated daily task for children we work with.

Not only does a child need to have oral motor support, they must also have good breath support to successfully navigate nutritious food. If we did not master the newborn rhythm of suck/swallow/breathe, we may fear choking. We may not be accepting of foods that we can't swallow quickly. We might stuff our cheeks and eat quickly so that we can catch our breath again.

When a child comes into my clinic as a loud and fast talker, I wonder about breath support. In the book, *The Connected Parent*, Lisa Qualls gives great advice for co-regulating with a child with the words, "Match my voice" when the child is a loud talker. It's a beautiful way to bring mindfulness and connection. But if the child does not have good abdominal support and lung capacity, this will be very difficult for them to accomplish. They may **want** to connect and co-regulate with you, but lack the skill to do so.

As an experiment, position your body as if you are doing a sit-up crunch while sitting in your chair. Try and take a deep breath. You should notice that your lung capacity is limited. When a child only has a short burst of air and lots to say, they will speak quickly to get their words out. A compensation position for this is to pull the shoulders up to stabilize the ribcage. This position will further increase the pitch of the vocals and sound louder. When we have good stabilizing core muscles, we are better able to oxygenate our blood to our brain to think more clearly as well as regulate our vocal pitch, tone, and word capacity. A simple Google search for singing and vocal exercises could reveal some really fun ways to increase breath support and decrease the volume and rate of the high-pitched fast talker.

Tips for the Loud Talker

- Swimming, blowing feathers or bubbles, and other things that require breath support.
- Teach core exercises to stabilize the rib cage.
- Make eye contact if comfortable and get down on the child's eye level to truly "listen" to them.
- Consider background noise, and if you can, move the child to a quieter area.
- Lower your own voice to a whisper. The child might mirror you.
- Speak in an accent. It is interesting and can promote focus because of the novelty.
- Respectfully repeat what the child says so they feel heard. Often, children will repeat loudly when they feel ignored.
- Be mindful of background noise. Children might compensate with a louder volume if they feel they must project over environmental noise.

Even if a child has good oral motor skill and breath support, taste can influence the acceptance of foods. Taste has aspects such as salty, sweet, sour, and spicy. Much of the preferences for these also rely heavily on cultural exposure and relationships. Certain aspects will invoke certain emotions, too. Sweet and salty hit the reward center of the brain while sour and spicy stimulate the autonomic nervous system and cause reflexive reactions such as sweating and lip puckering. Chewy food stimulates the proprioceptive system and can be calming. The sporadic, arrhythmic quality of crunchy food can be alerting. Because of this, we can influence the arousal state (calm vs. alert) depending upon what foods we offer.

As we look at therapeutic intervention for the gustatory sense, relationship is key, but there are some sensory-based strategies that might prove helpful. First and foremost, set the scene. Two exercises at feeding conferences that I found to be very valuable were setting the scene and building empathy.

The first exercise is to close your eyes and think of the best meal of your life. What comes to mind? Is it the actual food? Or do you see the lighting? Do you see people you love? Do you hear something in the background, soft music or laughter? Chances are, you are not alone. I'm guessing maybe something was being celebrated. Now, imagine if someone sat down next to you in that moment and started counting your bites. What if they started to criticize your portions or remind you how unhealthy something is? Would that change the meal for you? Earlier, I mentioned

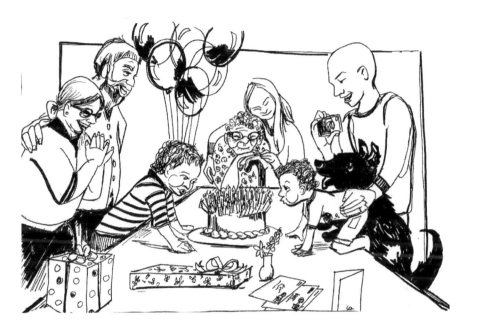

behaviors or habits that need therapy versus things that wouldn't prevent you from getting a second date. If your first date criticized everything about your plate or counted your bites, I'm guessing you wouldn't be too excited about a second date with that person. So don't be that person. Do the things you can to make a meal pleasant and relational. Use fun dishes. Get dishes that prevent food from touching if that helps. Always have at least one food item that the child consistently eats. If you told your date that you hated wild game and they served you nothing but various types of deer and bison, I'm guessing you wouldn't feel heard or valued. You might not want to share more meals with that person.

When dealing with food issues with a child, set the scene

with lighting, sounds, and the overall ambience in mind, then serve the food and let it be. If they don't eat, offer healthy choices at later times. As much as you can, make the meal about nurturing over nutrition. This is one of the reasons I suggest that "feeding therapy" happen outside of family mealtime. If you want to try strategies of taking small bites or slowly introducing new foods, it might be best to do that during a time when the child is not tired or there isn't the pressure of other family members watching them struggle. You could be playful with food in the bathtub or introduce new foods at a fun picnic where the consumption is optional. Allow the child to help prepare the food to gain exposure without the pressure of having to consume it. Experiment with different textures, keeping in mind that foods that stick together are easier to swallow.

Some children lack oral awareness and have difficulty perceiving the food inside their mouth. By adding spice or changing the temperature at which we offer the food, we increase the amount of information for them to process. For some children who are "seekers" and desire more input, these strategies can help them understand where the food is in their mouth and how to manage it. For other children, bland food is easier because they may be overwhelmed by too much stimulation. While most children who tend toward an overly alert state seek more input, it is best to view each child individually and uniquely each time you choose which type of food to present.

The next exercise is for empathy. One of the most

informative things I have done was to be blindfolded while a colleague fed me applesauce, pudding, and cottage cheese. It was incredibly eye opening. The exercise really emphasized for me how speed of food introduction, explanation of what I'm about to receive, and spoon placement affected my experience. It forced me to understand how intimate feeding someone is and helped me appreciate the value in communication and connection.

Much of our sense of taste is related not only to consistency and flavor, but also smell. When a food is heated, the moisture begins to evaporate and the smells reach our nasal passages, contributing to our sense of taste. For this reason, consider temperature as another variable to adjust when working to improve eating habits.

It is understood in the food industry that the scents of butter, bread, and sugar will increase our hunger. Restaurants commonly bring warm, fresh bread to the table to stimulate our hunger and encourage us to order more food than we may have otherwise. One trick I recall from working in an assisted living facility was to pop buttered popcorn as a snack before dinner time. Since the sense of taste diminishes with age, many of the residents didn't get enough calories. We discovered that the buttery smell of the popcorn and using orange dishes (a visual hunger stimulus), our residents' food intake increased.

Recalling the success of this practice, I once took my daughter to a Scentsy candle party and asked her to identify which candle smell made her hungry. She proudly proclaimed "linen sheets" was the scent that made her mouth water. So, each night about twenty minutes before dinner, I would burn that scented wax. Oddly enough, it worked. Her caloric intake was greater on the days we warmed wax that smelled like linen sheets.

Much of our experience of taste actually comes from smell. Think back to times when you've had a cold or sinus infection. It's likely the decreased ability to smell your food impacted your enjoyment of it. We can also use this to our advantage. Considering that warmed food releases moisture that gives it a stronger smell, cold smoothies can help get nutrition into children that are over-sensitive to smells. I don't hide things in a smoothie; that's a quick way to lose trust and have a child potentially refuse the few foods they are willing to eat. But I've observed that when I blend things into a smooth, thick, frosty, and "bolusable" formula, the child can swallow it easily. Furthermore, the cold temperature provides extra sensory input for the child to understand how the smoothie is moving in their mouth and adding a lid with a straw further decreases the smell so that the spinach (or whatever may be in there) doesn't taste as "green."

For some children, food has replaced relationship or they lack the interoception to know when they are full. I know I am often guilty of "eating my emotions." Without the cues of lighting, sounds, and other things that make mealtime a multi-sensory experience, we often turn to carb-rich, sugary foods. These foods give us a serotonin boost to improve our mood instantly and a sugar rush to increase our alert level when we are bored or tired. Unfortunately, this boost is short lived, addictive, and non-sustaining. Yet, it is sometimes culturally how we express love.

One of my favorite memories of my Grandma Carolyn is her cookie baking. Those who know me personally have likely had one of Grandma Carolyn's cookies. I love to bake them to show my love. Because that's how Grandma showed me love. My children laugh at how I retell a common interaction of my youth with Grandma Carolyn. She would pat my chubby thigh and say, "Mmmmmm mmmmmm mmmmmm. Look at these thick thighs." Then there would be an uncomfortable pause. Then she would say, "Here. Have a cookie." She was the 1946 Miss Indiana and competed in the Miss America pageant. She had a beauty like Marilyn Monroe and held onto her fashion and vanity into her nineties. And she loved her cookies. It was a delicious contradiction of my heritage. I don't think I'm alone. The aunts and grandmas seem to get away with telling us things that would horrify us if told by other family members. But that yummy food is a great emotional buffer. Romantic comedies are full of young girls pouring their heartache into a pint of ice cream. Many people find food to be a comfort they aren't able to receive from the caregiver. So, they find it in a carton.

Some children I work with are fearful of starvation. When their neural connections were forming, their needs were not consistently met. These children sometimes hoard or hide food to make sure it will be available for them. In the past, a common response was for the caregiver to lock the food up, which can signal to the child that they are unworthy of the nurture and nutrition provided by food. A better option is to allow them to hoard food but work within the relationship to find ways that don't cause sanitation issues. Instead of hoarding bananas, maybe they can have a basket of wrapped granola bars in their room.

Hydration is another common concern for children who have experienced adversity. Poor hydration can lead to electrolyte imbalances. If the body chemistry is not optimal, the neural synapses will not function optimally either. With some clients, adding a sport drink every other day has made a significant difference in their mood and sleep. Whenever I recommend any type of vitamin or supplement, I make sure the caregivers also consult with their physician or a nutrition specialist. I will often suggest an over-the-counter product to be used for up to a week. If it is found to be helpful, I request that they follow up with someone licensed to advise them on the use of supplements.

Children with poor interoception may not realize they are thirsty. Dehydration is a common presentation with many of my clients. As we discussed earlier, water is a consistency that children with less mature feeding skills can choke on. Fizzy sodas, smoothies, and sugar-filled drinks provide more input to the senses and are actually easier to swallow for many children. Of course, these sugary, caffeinated drinks don't help with hydration and raise additional concerns.

One thing I have found to be helpful is to allow the child to drink from a straw. In addition to blocking some of the smell a straw places the neck in a forward flexed position, a much easier position for swallowing.

I'm continually baffled when I see a caregiver trying to teach a child to swallow something as they stand above them, requiring the child to look up. As an experiment, take a sip of a beverage. Tilt your head back with your eyes to the ceiling. Now try and swallow. It is anatomically very challenging. Next, take that same sip and flex your head forward with your eyes to your belly button. Often, the fluid simply rolls back and down in that anatomical position.

While the gustatory sense seems pretty straightforward, it becomes more complicated when viewed through the lens of early trauma, and when we consider the psychological associations that are formed with the sense of taste. The interplay of taste with interoception complicates things further. Stress can upset the stomach, an overstimulated vestibular system can make us feel nauseous, and a multitude of other internal sensations can interfere with eating. Too often, these feelings make feeding very difficult for children, and they miss out on the healthy, nutritious food that will ultimately nourish them. Hopefully this chapter has given you some "food for thought," as you consider how the sense of taste goes further than the tip of your tongue.

As we discuss individual senses, it is important to note that not all challenges with the senses are related to trauma or relationship. If a limb is amputated, there could be phantom limb sensations. If a child requires glasses or a hearing aid, these are often anatomical, medical conditions. Of course, medical trauma (car wreck, burn, head trauma) could contribute to sensory processing issues. Some sensory issues have a genetic or medical component and require a more medical approach. While these connection strategies will be helpful, I encourage the reader to reach beyond these suggestions when necessary. The gustatory sense can be affected by medical conditions including food allergies, Crohn's disease, reflux, celiac disease, irritable bowel disease, and others. These conditions require medical intervention beyond what is being covered in this text.

Helpful Tips for Picky Eaters

- NEVER force a food on a child.
- Allow a "no thank you" plate where the child can remove the food if needed. Control will help with later acceptance.
- Recognize that poor nutrition with good connection is better than good nutrition with poor connection. Good connection will foster better nutrition over time.
- Recognize that most children are picky as part of normal development. They usually eat better around age twelve.
- Use vitamins blended into cold shakes with straws

to help increase nutritional intake.

- Allow healthy snacks for food security. Make them easily available and easy to transport.
- Engage with the child in food prep, planning, shopping, mixing, and cooking.
- Freeze food so that has a different feel and smell.
- A pudding consistency is easiest to swallow if a child has poor oral motor skills.
- Foods that stick together (purees, mashed potatoes, oatmeal,) are less likely to cause choking than foods that scatter in the mouth (carrots, meats, salads).
- Allow food art and food sensory exploration.
- Add spices to increase the sensory information.
- Play with textures, temperatures, and tastes.
- Set aside time for food exploration separate from mealtime. Allow the child to display terrible table manners and even spit the food out. Be PLAYFUL during this time.
- Invest in the plate separator, shovel spoon, special cup. Find ways to make mealtime FUN.
- Do not pick family mealtime to count bites or monitor food intake. Family meals should be focused on connection, not content. Work on food content during the child's best time of day (often right before lunch).

OLFACTORY: THE SENSE OF SMELL

The sense of smell is interpreted in the amygdala and is strongly connected to emotion and memory. Smell is also very connected to heritage. Foods from different cultures have different smells and can even affect the smells of our bodies. Think about how a person smells after eating a lot of garlic, onions, curry, or other spices. If these foods are part of your heritage, they are more likely to be familiar and comforting, when literally emanating from someone's pores. Different areas of the world also have different smells. The salty, fishy ocean smells different from a desert or the rainforest. The example of my "monkey perfume" in the beginning of this book is just another example of how smells and familiarity influence our attachments and relationships.

Memory and smell are intertwined to help ensure our survival. Studies show that pheromones (the smell of hormones involved with reproductive functions) are difficult to detect consciously but are interpreted by the olfactory sense and influence dating behavior, thereby maintaining the survival of our species and influencing our partner choices. Memory and smell also work together to protect us from danger. When we smell smoke, our arousal level increases. Our eyes become more focused and our blood pumps to prepare us to get away. When food smells rotten, our stomach tightens and our esophagus constricts, helping to prevent us from consuming something that might harm us.

At the time of this writing, COVID-19 has been making the rounds through our family's friend group. Many of them say the loss of taste and smell has decreased their quality of life and the pleasure they take in food. One of my friends worries now that she won't smell a fire. She doesn't know when food is rotten or if dinner is burning. This concern has led to more anxiety and prompted her to ask more questions of those around her. She is also relying more heavily on her other senses. The experience has given her greater empathy for children whose senses don't relay accurate information.

Smell can be primitive and polarizing. It can bring great calm with familiar or pleasing scents and great alarm with unfamiliar or pungent scents. When considering childhood trauma, it is important to consider what smells might have been familiar to the child. What scents were paired with nurture? What scents were paired with neglect? A caregiver who smoked marijuana may have been very calm and nurturing during the times when the smoke was present, so its smell might be associated with those feelings. Conversely, a caregiver who smoked marijuana may have been neglectful during those times, forgetting to feed, change, or attend to the child. In that case, the small would be associated with lonely, uncomfortable feelings. Once again, our past experiences and current expectations will greatly influence our sensory preferences.

In my clinical experience, I have found some patterns that might be helpful as caregivers consider smell as part of a sensory experience. First, a caution: A respected colleague once helped me understand the effects of synthetic scents and natural scents. She explained that when vendors like Yankee Candle manufacture their scented candles, they add a chemical binder that clings to nasal hair receptors and causes the scent to linger in the nasal cavity. Thus, the scent stays with a person for several minutes after the stimulation is removed. My colleague offered this information as a possible explanation for why people sometimes get headaches or have adverse reactions to synthetically-scented products, but tolerate naturally-derived oils and scents. For this reason, you may want to avoid artificial scents in your treatments.

When I worked with autism, I often encountered children with a heightened sense of smell. They seemed to react very strongly to the odor of the school's cleaning products and even the natural odors of food in the cafeteria. And yet, their own body odor seemed pleasing to them. If you've ever seen the "Super Star" skits on *Saturday Night Live*, you may have a good visual of armpit smells in your mind. As unhygienic as this seems, for some people, the lure of the personal scent is strong.

I observed that teachers' smells, such as coffee breath, strong perfume, hair products, etc., could sometimes trigger strong "shutdown" reactions in students, but that other olfactory information could be used to support calming and connection. I recall that the Victoria's Secret Vanilla Lace scent, in particular, seemed to have a calming effect when used as a lotion. As a young therapist, I went against the advice of my mentors to not use any scented products and put just a little on my wrists. Children who typically pulled away and resisted physical contact would often smooth their bodies up against mine to be closer. I would feel them relax as they inhaled close to my wrists. Once again, I was "one of them." Not only did the scent help calm the children, but it also helped me, as we navigated together through the smells of the cafeteria and the perfumes and coffee breath of their well-intended teachers.

Oils on the wrist also became a much-appreciated strategy with some of the aides I worked with. We had a particularly gassy child one year, and the air quality became questionable at times. Once the aides started putting citrus oil on their wrists, students' eyes began to sparkle a bit more clearly through the cloudy aroma. Since the classroom had two aides who shared the oil, they also had the relational buffer of a buddy. They were able to knowingly smile at one another and sniff their wrists in relational community, which helped build resilience against the innocent but odiferous onslaught to their noses.

Another trick I learned from a seasoned therapist in one of my courses was to simply keep an orange at my desk. This therapist noticed that at around three p.m., which is a common time for a coffee or tea break, she would get a bit sleepy. As she sat down to complete her documentation toward the end of the day, she would rub the orange between her palms. This rubbing released the orange oil through the peel, and the scent would alert as much as a cup of coffee or tea.

Smell is a strong sense. But it is an easy one to experiment with, when striving toward the just-right environment. Absent any chemical modifications, once a smell stimulus is removed, the effects don't tend to be long lasting. Smell can be effective for a quick response, which also promotes quick positive changes in alert or calm arousal states.

I am always amused by our inherent desire to share a bad smell or taste. "Does this smell rotten to you? This is so gross. Taste it!" These seem like weird things to say until we frame them in the context of a relationship. On the surface we are saying, "Here, taste/smell this awful thing." But on a deeper level, we are really asking for a buddy to match our momentary over-alert arousal state and help us come back to calm, within the context of the relationship. This kind of shared social interaction helps make memories and gives us more stories for that future campfire together.

Tactile: The Sense of Touch

As we discussed in the proprioceptive section, touch is more than skin deep. Most discussions of touch only scratch the surface.

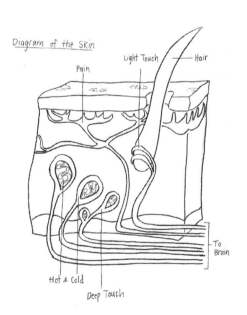

The science of the tactile system goes far beyond light touch or deep touch. Each sensory receptor has its own nerve path, which is interpreted differently in the brain. Hair follicles are easily stimulated and feel vibration in the air around a person. Deep touch receptors are deeper in the skin and require more force to stimulate.

In general, light touch and more extreme temperature tend to alert us, while deep touch and neutral temperatures tend to calm us. As with smell, the tactile system is anatomically designed for protection but is influenced by relational connection. An interesting point to consider about touch is the difference between *known touch* and *unknown touch*. For example, it is physically impossible to tickle yourself. The element of surprise simply isn't there once you engage the cortex to motor-plan the act of touching yourself. This lack of surprise helps us tolerate touch from caregivers and people in our immediate social circle. Because we have a history with these people, we have had the repeated relational experiences that help us develop deep neural pathways to normalize that person's safe touch on our bodies. While we can make generalizations about touch, we should always consider relationship and interpretation of previous experiences.

Neurologically, light touch is alerting. But for some children, the light touch of a caregiver on their back at bedtime is calming. Children may calm to this input for two reasons. One, the caregiver has lovingly repeated that rhythmic, repetitive, relational touch and the child has habituated or paired that stimulus with deep nurture and connection. Two, the child doesn't register tactile input well unless it is amplified. Therefore, that alerting touch helps them actually feel their body as they attempt to calm.

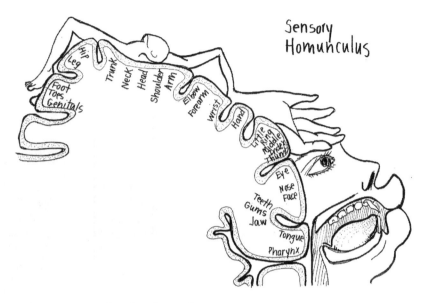

Sensory Homunculus

As a general rule, I tend to recommend not tickling at bedtime unless there is a strong relational, deep touch, and proprioceptive component to the stimulation.

Another point of anatomical interest is the distribution of touch receptors throughout our body. When we look at the cortical homunculus, we see that not all body parts get equal representation. There are significantly more touch receptors in the hands, lips, genitalia, and back of the neck, mainly to support safety, procreation, and fine-motor dexterity. The more nerve receptors per square inch of skin, the more information the brain has to interpret tactile sensations. This understanding of tactile receptor distribution is one reason I support CapeAble weighted products. Many of the weighted products on the market, or ones made by well-intended do-it-yourselfers, contain beads or other weighted particles contained in large spaces. As a seamstress, I've made my share of homemade weighted items. It is truly difficult to make small compartments that hold those little beads in place. When CapeAble founder Marna Pancheo developed the SmartWeight™ technology that allowed her industrial machines to sew two-inch compartments for the beads, she gained the benefit of anatomical integrity. Since most areas of skin that are covered by a weighted blanket contain sensory receptors every two inches, her beads maintain their pressure more therapeutically. Other weighted items can slip and slide over the nerve sensors and mimic the feeling of someone or something moving across the skin, which is a very alerting sensation for most people.

As occupational therapists, we study a skill called *stereognosis*. This is the ability to identify an object based on feeling without looking at it. It is how we identify coins on the inside of our pockets or know which key to use without having to rely on our vision. Thinking of the nerve distribution, consider how much easier it is to distinguish between a nickel and a penny held in your hand, versus a nickel and a penny placed on your forearm. For children whose tactile system does not have sufficient ability to receive, interpret, or respond to sensation, their experience of holding a pencil or spoon may be experienced as if it was placed on their forearm: They struggle to understand its position on their body and how to grasp and utilize it appropriately.

As we consider adverse experiences and how they

shape our preferences, we gain a better understanding of why some children develop tactile defensiveness or touch aversion. Our skin is considered our largest organ, and it is the most easily accessible to stimulate. Children with tactile defensiveness or aversion to touch have trouble protecting themselves against a perceived onslaught of unwanted stimulation. Tags bother these children because they stimulate areas of the body that have the most sensory receptors. Hugs are rejected because they feel restricting or too intense. Paint and food sauces can't be tolerated because the trickle feeling on the skin is simply too intense. Connection attempts such as holding hands or rubbing of the back are too sporadic to be calming for some children.

The tongue also contains tactile receptors, leading some tactile-aversive children to strictly regulate food textures. In a healthy, nurturing relationship, the caregiver has given the baby many repeated neural experiences of being caressed as they were fed and gazed upon. They received these little bursts of alert followed by the proprioceptive, relational calm. In many of the children I work with, this paired learning never took place. For them, these caresses may be perceived as light touch or pain responses that need to be rubbed away or run from. Conversely, some children have experienced so much adverse touch that their bodies have habituated to the stimulus and simply stopped responding to it. Habituation is very common with the skin. For example, if you've put on uncomfortable socks, you know that after a few minutes, you get used to the sensation.

That's habituation, your body deciding these socks aren't going to kill you and ceasing to interpret the sensation of the socks against your skin. This habituation happens even more readily when it is paired with deep touch, such as snug-fitting shoes.

Some children are kept very clean, and they don't get to experience running through the woods with their friends, giggling together as they jump off rocks into springy moss, or touch prickly pinecones and feathery ferns. Many modern children simply haven't had the necessary relational repetition to build a resilient tactile system. Other children received too much uncomfortable tactile stimulation without the buffer of relational repair. These children may experience sensory-system shutdown and may become constant tactile seekers who need to feel EVERYTHING. In either case, some therapists find a technique called the Wilbarger Deep Touch Protocol to be helpful. Simply put, this protocol uses a specialized scrub brush that stimulates the tactile system every two hours and then pairs it with the relational deep touch input that helps the body "organize" the information and no longer perceive it as a threat. I've taken the training for this approach twice and I've seen it work wonders for many children, including my own.

While the actual protocol is designed to be administered only by trained professionals, I've had caregivers get results by simply rubbing a washcloth on their child while pairing the stimulus with deep touch input in a connected, relational way. I've not done any studies to compare the two methods. For those with ongoing, function-limiting tactile irregularities, it may be worth seeking an occupational therapist or other trained professional to assist. The washcloth method would fall into the "can't hurt, might help" category, especially if used as a normal part of bath time. The bathtub washcloth process is pretty tried and true and although many children may have thought they would die from a good scrub, I know of no known actual cases of death by a nurturing bath time. I believe the chances of harm decrease even more when they are wrapped in a warm towel and told a sweet bedtime story at the end of the experience.

The perception of temperature is another widely variable sensory experience. Children with sensory differences often wear clothing that doesn't match the weather. But it can be tricky to understand why. Is the child avoiding long sleeves to reduce the tactile sensation of fabric against their arms? Or are they actually seeking more input from the cold air to help them feel and experience their bodies? These questions need to be considered, but simple sensory checklists can be confusing. Both examples lead to an observation of "avoids long sleeves." But one child seeks more input and the other is avoiding it. These checklists can help us organize our observations, but they can't give easy scoring results. Again, the sensory system does not happen in isolation. The goal is to look for patterns within these checklists rather than "if, then" diagnostics. A simple checklist I recommend is by Lindsey Biel, OTR/L, and can be found through her website as well as on my Trauma Informed OT Pinterest board. I'll introduce my own tool that I use for sensory that I use for sensory activity recommendations, KALMAR, later in this book.

AUDITORY: THE SENSE OF SOUND

Music is said to calm the savage soul. When we hear sounds, our reaction is immediate. Sound is a powerful therapeutic tool, and therapists can use it to help calm or alert a child. Fast and arrhythmic music tends to be alerting, while slow and rhythmic music tends to be calming. When I want to match a child's arousal state for connection, music and rhythm are often my go-to therapeutic techniques. I will match their rhythm in the bounce of my feet. I might tap my leg, clap my hands, or even thump on a drum if I have one. By matching their movement with an auditory stimulus, I am sending a signal of connection.

In the Therapeutic Listening course I took from Sheila Frick, OTR, I learned that she created music tracts that, simply put, filter the various frequencies. This filtering helps exercise and train the inner ear muscles, which move in reaction to sound and provide auditory input to our brain. Many modified music courses are several days long, and I'm not trained to actually teach them. So, I will keep this text within my experience, with the goal of providing you simple strategies that "can't hurt, might help."

My first introduction to therapeutic music was with a boy who had received several vaccinations during a time when his immune system was already fighting something.

I am not anti-vax. But I am pro spreading the vaccines out and considering each individual's immune system. I think vaccines are vital to keeping our community safe, and both of my children are fully vaccinated. As I type this, I'm looking forward to my first COVID-19 vaccine. I simply spread vaccines out across doctor visits, and I don't give vaccines when my child appears to already be fighting something.

My little client experienced the perfect storm of his underlying sensitivity, an acute infection, and multiple vaccines at once. It was the first time I saw what I would consider a "vaccine reaction." It definitely had an impact for me to be so close to it.

While treating this child, I did all the "can't hurt, might help" things I could think of. I gave mom intense home programming for reflex integration. We were stimulating both sides of his brain simultaneously trying to get things to fire and wire back together. He was losing language, he was losing muscle tone, he seemed to be losing nervous system function and myelation quickly.

At the time, my daughter was using a therapeutic listening program that one of my colleagues who was treating her had prescribed for us. So I had that one CD at home at the time. As I often do, I prayed for the sweet boy who was my current puzzle before I went to bed one night. In what I believe was divine intervention, I woke up from a dream where the boy was wearing my child's headphones. I figured it couldn't hurt, might even help. So, the next day, we put the headphones on him using my daughter's therapeutic music. It was a miraculous transformation. In my previous ten years of therapy in both inpatient and outpatient treatment of adults and children, I had never seen such a quick positive result. He sat up straight and started talking within about twenty minutes.

My mind was blown. I sent my headphones home with the mom that day and he continued to make progress. At the time, I didn't have the budget for the training myself and there were no courses in my area. So, I googled things. I found the man who wrote the EASe CDs and explained to him what I had seen and asked if he had any resources. He had a wealth of information and even sent me a few new CDs to try. He has developed some really cool products that are cost-effective and he explains things very thoroughly. For more information, I highly recommend https://audioforge. net/. He has even developed an app that will change the BPM (beats per minute) of the music on your phone. *Tempo Magic* is an older app that I have had success with as well.

I have concluded that most auditory sensitivity can be helped by exercising the inner ear muscles, which these modified music programs are designed to do. I have found that they either work quickly and well, or not at all. I once prescribed modified music for a child. I first gave mom the headphones, so she could hear what her child was hearing. Almost immediately, the mom closed her eyes and started making "intimate" sounds. It was comically uncomfortable to witness. After she composed herself, she agreed that the music could potentially trigger strong emotional reactions.

Other children show no response at all. When new therapists or parents ask my opinion on using therapeutic music with a specific child, I often introduce them to the less expensive *EASe app*. If a child reacts positively, I then encourage them to explore the more expensive options and help them find a trained therapist to help. For therapists who may be trained and still feel underqualified, I recommend the *EASe* app audioforge website, http://blog.audioforge.org/2012/12/transcript-of-ease-lecture.html

If you purchase the inexpensive *EASe* app, there are full instructions in the manual that I have found to be more helpful than any course I have taken.

The modified music programs are powerful for children whose auditory system developed atypically due to adverse experience, trauma, or other conditions. But almost anyone responds to rhythm, which is part of our human experience across the lifespan. Rhythm and rhythmic sounds can be experienced through weather, biological functions, communication, artistic expression, and even the vibration of the earth itself. Rhythmic sounds of the heartbeat, swooshing amniotic fluid, and outside noises are some of the first sensory input we "feel" in utero.

My friend Michael Remole, MA LCPC, taught me that horses will match heartbeats up to twelve feet away. This is one reason why equine-assisted therapy can be so powerful. Horses have large thumping hearts that a person can feel as they co-regulate with the horse. Studies show that if we are stimulated with rhythmic proprioceptive input such as the horse heartbeat, tapping, drumming, or heavy bass music, our heartbeat will adjust to synchronize. I've even had success with the rhythm of my breath. A college girlfriend once told me the easiest way to "catch a date" was to wear lipstick and match my date's breath rate as I cuddled in close. I'm not saying this is scientifically sound. But I will say I didn't lack for dates in college.

There are various theories relating to arousal-level adjustment. Some involve a top-down approach, in which a client uses cognitive ideas to lower a heart rate. Others involve a bottom-up approach, in which a person focuses on breath and physical movement to change heart rate. Physicians even prescribe blood pressure medication at times for people who have explosive "alert" tendencies. The theory behind this is to pharmaceutically lower the blood pressure and heart rate, to help the rest of the body to calm. In my NMT studies, there is growing evidence of bottom-up calming strategies, or bottom-up regulation.

If a person can identify that their arousal level is high, they can engage, within the context of relationship, in somatosensory activities (bottom-up) that will lower the arousal level. Many of these techniques involve rhythmic, repetitive, relational activities. Music fits these categories perfectly. Music is an actual sound wave. We both hear and feel it. The more bass present, the more proprioception we encounter.

Music also connects people together, so our heartbeats shift within the context of relationship when we listen to music together. If our heartbeats match, our arousal levels begin to match, and we can then enter a co-regulated and connected state. Do you have an "our song" or a "my jam" that you share with someone? That sharing is once again a relationship. Teenagers often co-regulate with music. Interestingly, the higher our heartbeat, the higher the tempo we prefer. We want to be matched on that brainstem level. Since children and teens have higher resting heart beats than most adults, most children and teenagers prefer faster tempo music. And yet, a little AC/DC can bring my generation off the couch as we nostalgically transport ourselves back to our youth. People with tendencies toward hyperactivity will also prefer faster tempo music. Because it feels better when our arousal level is matched.

So how do we use tempo therapeutically? Just like so many other things, the key to auditory intervention is subtle relational connection. We meet the individual where their current heartbeat sits. If they are hyperactive, we are going to play more upbeat, strong bass music to match them. Then, we can create playlists to gradually bring them back down. In settings where a group may be moving from an outside recess activity into a quiet activity, a transitional cadence can be helpful. As you line up to walk through the hall, meet the cadence of the outside BPM and then slowly bring the group down to the desired cadence as you approach the next room. *Tempo Magic* and the *Audio Step* app can be very useful tools for this strategy.

The impact of heart rate on our arousal level is the premise behind targeted playlists. There is music for studying, for relaxing, for running, for cleaning, etc. Music streaming companies like Spotify and Pandora have written algorithms that measure the BPM and select songs based on features such as tempo, genre, or historical timelines. In general, calming activities such as relaxing with a favorite pet or listening to ocean waves in a hammock will be in the forty to sixty BPM category. Quiet alert activities such as creating art or desk work will be in the sixty to eighty BPM range while fast paced, energetic activities will be eighty to 110 BPM. Exercise and cardio type activities will be in the 110-200 BPM range.

Music is also relational because it often tells a story. Country and folk songs, especially, tell a relatable tale for an audience. Even music without words can convey different feelings. I remember when a music teacher in middle school played a film without any music. It was so bizarre, and it made me much more aware of how filmmakers use musical scoring to convey the emotional tone of the story. While I'm not musically gifted myself, I do feel the influence of music on my emotions and mood when listening.

Music also helps us remember things. Putting lists to a rhythm increases your ability to remember them. I remember singing the theme song to the television show *Happy Days* to recall the days of the week and counting from one to twe-e-e-e-eelve with *Sesame Street*. Different cultures and generations create anthems to remember things as well. The sixties were full of war songs. People often express cultural emotion and feelings through song. Our unique voices even convey rhythm, pitch, vibration, and such.

Different sounds and types of speech evoke different emotions and activate different parts of the brain. For example, singing and speech do not originate in the same portion of the brain. I've had a few patients who could sing after a stroke but they could not talk. When I worked in an outpatient surgical recovery room during high school, a nurse trained me to lower my tone when I spoke with sleepy patients as they began to wake up. When I used my high-pitched cheerleader voice, I got very little response.

She taught me to go lower and speak from deep in my chest. It was much more effective. I found this trick handy later, when I began to work with children who had autism. Sometimes, simply lowering my voice or adding a sing-song pattern would help me communicate with these students more effectively. As we age, our voice patterns change, and our hearing preferences change as well. Young children have higher heart rates, move faster, have a faster "rhythm," and prefer a higher-pitched tone. Some people start to favor lower tones as they age.

When we consider the auditory processing of children who have experienced adversity, it is important to once again consider what their environment was like when they were developing these skills. Did they receive rich language, nursery rhymes, lullabies, and enthusiastic encouragement paired with calming deep touch input? Or did they experience sporadic yelling, alarms, high-pitched screaming, and other auditorily offensive input? Did they have any auditory input at all? All of these early experiences will shape their preferences and how they interpret future "background music."

Helpful Tips for Auditory Sensitivity

- Remember that young children respond more to high-pitched voices while adults respond more to low-pitched voices.
- Consult with an occupational therapist, speech therapist, or other provider who is knowledgeable in auditory processing and auditory/listening/

music therapies.

- When an individual screams, the stapedius muscle inside the ear activates and dampens the noise to the screamer. For some children, a scream is an effective way to block out auditory stimulation.
- When a child covers their ears, they may not be trying to ignore you. It may be a coping mechanism to block out external stimulation. Reframing this behavior can help us respond more empathetically.
- When engaging in listening therapies, wireless headphones allow more freedom of movement.
- Noise cancelling headphones not only decrease the amount of auditory sensation being interpreted, they provide proprioceptive input to both sides of the body through the skull's parietal bones. I've noticed a calming response to this input even when the gentle pressure is provided with my hands without the headphones.
- A sweatshirt hoodie or stocking cap can be an effective way to decrease auditory stimulation for children who are unable to tolerate headphones.
- When children make frequent guttural noises (clearing the throat/grunting), consider whether there may be dysfunction in the digestive tract or allergies. I have found that some children who make these noises have a medical diagnosis of GERD or post-nasal drip. Antacids, over-the-counter allergy medications, and prescription medications have

made significant improvements in these issues for many of my personal clients.

VISION: THE SENSE OF SIGHT

While proprioception is the relational sense and the vestibular sense is the influential sense, vision is the sense that I find most professionals overlook when working with children who have experienced trauma. I've not kept formal documentation on this issue, but anecdotally, it seems that

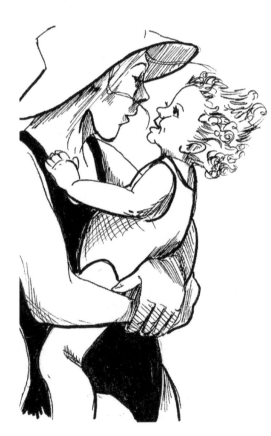

a high number of the children I work with who experienced early trauma or neglect also have difficulty with their eye muscles. Visual acuity is easily tested with the simple eye charts in the pediatrician office. But oculomotor skills, or the use of eye muscles, are often overlooked in simple screenings When an infant is born, they only see clearly for a range of ten to twelve inches in front of them. This is perfect for attachment. Imagine how many opportunities the infant has to gaze into their mother's face as they breastfeed? It's like the entire rest of the world is blurred aside from their mother's face and loving gaze. Bottle-feeding moms should be encouraged to position their babies similarly to breast-feeding moms for this reason. As the baby matures, their visual field gets wider, and they begin to see more colors and patterns.

Around the age of three months, the baby will start to follow objects at a greater distance than twelve inches. Around six months, the baby will begin to reach for objects close to them. At nine months, a big jump occurs in the visual system, often correlating with when the baby starts to crawl. As the baby is on all fours, there is a bone in the base of the skull that prevents the head from going backwards too far. Because of this, the head cannot extend to place the eyes towards the ceiling. It is during this stage of development and learning to navigate the world in the crawling (four-point) position that the eye muscles get a huge workout. Since the skull becomes fixed in this position, the eye muscles must work hard to take in all the visual input in the environment. These tiny eye muscles are still muscles. Muscles get stronger and more proficient and develop muscle memory when they are used repeatedly.

The rhythmic pattern of the crawl also aids in the development of this input. As the baby crawls under tables, around couches, and up and down hallways, the eyes are constantly scanning and strengthening. This is one reason why tummy time and crawling are such important developmental skills. Now consider how early trauma and adverse experience may impact this critical window of development for the visual system. If a child does not experience a loving gaze or playful peekaboo games, they don't develop those strong visual attachments. If they are left in a crib or car seat all the time, those muscles never develop to be strong and efficient. This underdevelopment can cause difficulty later with reading, scanning a room, eye-hand coordination, and many other foundational and functional skills.

Our visual system is also connected to our emotional responses. Our eyes physically **weep** when we are sad. The eyes are the windows to the soul. We get a "look in our eye" that others who are perceptive can understand and interpret. Being "seen" is a big deal for little children. A great place to see this in action is a playground or swimming pool. The gleeful squeals of "Watch this! Look at me! Did you see that?" all indicate our need to be seen.

On a more mechanical level, the eye muscles react to different emotions. I am a constant student of body language. Maybe because I have difficulty with reading people's facial cues and emotional tones, I have a keen interest in how the body moves. Although not entirely accurate, I find it interesting that people do tend to point their body towards people who make them comfortable. We flex forward when we are sad or disconnected. We extend when we are excited or welcoming. A secret I learned from a dear friend is to always wear lipstick and mascara, because the eyes and the

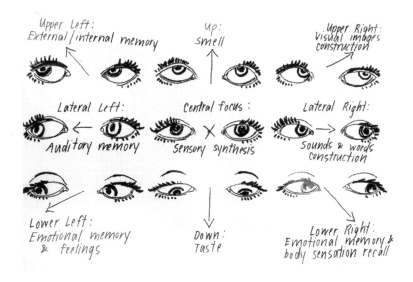

lips are the most powerful communicators. The eyes even move different directions based on feelings, memories, and thoughts.

I have noticed eye patterns and emotions within my own clinic. When a person is upset, they tend to look up. Sometimes this is paired with rhythmic waving of the hands in an effort to hold off tears. When we look up, we are less likely to cry. It is our way of trying to calm ourselves through body movements, a quick dissociation to bring our thinking brain back online. However, consider a child whose eye muscles did not get strong enough when they were a baby. This child tries to look up, but they end up extending their neck to compensate for the lack of stability in the eye muscles. This movement alerts the vestibular system that the head is falling backwards towards the ground. The vestibular system then sends out the alarm to protect the head. I see this so often clinically. The very thing the child does to self-calm ends up alerting them.

When I teach live courses, I often have participants pretend their eye muscles don't work and experience some of these movements. How much more alert are you if you look up toward the ceiling by extending your neck? How much more alert are you if your eyes don't move and you scan the room around you? Does this experiment increase your compassion for the child who prefers to always wear a hoodie or a ball cap? Do you see how that is actually helping them stay calm by decreasing the amount of peripheral vision they have to process? How does this change the way we view children who have experienced adversity? If they don't have typical physical skills or eye muscle control, are we expecting too much of them?

This lack of eye muscle development causes more engagement of the vestibular system as the child attempts to survey their surroundings. Consider what happens when a child walks into a room. With normal development, the child's head is relatively static/still and the eyes can glance around using the muscles to assess the visual input and see if there is anything that can be perceived as dangerous. For the child with weak eye muscles, however, the head once again compensates and becomes a swiveling axis upon the spinal cord. As we remember from the discussion of the vestibular system, this spinning movement is one of the most alerting movements for the vestibular sense.

For deeper understanding of these issues, it is important

to consider two types of vision, *focal vision* and *peripheral vision*. Focal vision is the calm vision. This is when the eyes converge at midline to help us read something directly in front of us or focus on something small and precise. Peripheral vision is away from the midline. This type of vision scans for things that might come at us quickly or otherwise be a threat. If someone tosses something your way that you aren't expecting, you use peripheral vision to quickly assess what it is, and whether you are in danger. Horses have very active peripheral vision and are considered prey animals, meaning they are often on the alert for danger. Sometimes their handlers will put on blinders so that the horse doesn't see the alerting visual input that would distract them from their goals/work. If we consider the example of scanning a room, we can see how the vestibular system is activated along with our peripheral visual system.

Sensory recommendations are always suggestions and not prescriptions, and it is important to consider the perspective of the person using the strategy. A child who has experienced adversity must feel a sense of control and safety with modifications. For example, a ball cap or hoodie can be used to help a child who feels safe but their peripheral vision is easily overstimulated. This simple modification could be very beneficial to decrease the distraction of a visually complex classroom environment. But, if a child is constantly scanning the room in an attempt to feel safe, I would not put a ball cap or hood on them to further limit their vision. They would consequently just move their neck even more in an attempt to scan for safety, thereby increasing their alerting vestibular input. When providing modifications, it is always important to communicate with the person and make sure you are not taking away a coping mechanism that they have developed in order to feel safe.

Once I understood how the visual system and weak eye muscles can affect arousal levels and can appear similar to ADHD and other diagnoses, I began to look more closely at the eye muscles of my clients. A simple, "Please try and keep your head still as you follow my finger" is an easy thing to add to any assessment. If they have to move their head to follow my finger, I know I need to work to strengthen those muscles. I've had a lot of success collaborating with vision therapists on several cases. *Eye Exerciser* is an app I've used with some success for mild cases. Eyecanlearn. com is another free online resource I have found beneficial for more information and free exercises.

The eyes are also connected to the vestibular system and autonomic arousal/brainstem function. When someone has a head injury or whiplash, medical personnel check for pupil dilation. "Pupils fixed and dilated" is a sign of a really poor brain injury prognosis. Pupils should react to light without any cognitive thought required. We can use this automatic function to our benefit. If someone is in an overly alert state, their pupils may dilate to prepare to take in more light and information. If we move the person to a brighter room, the pupils may constrict due to the extra light and it could help bring the person back into a state of calm. You can see the potential benefit of working with this system when you imagine a tantruming toddler who calms easily when taken outside in the sunlight. No matter our age, sometimes a change in lighting can help us calm down.

The brightness and focus of the lighting can be additional therapeutic tools. When I worked with people with traumatic brain injuries, they were often overwhelmed and distracted by sensory stimuli. To help facilitate physical rehab, I would carry a flashlight with a base. I used this as a spotlight. If I wanted the patient to do some finger, hand, or leg exercise, I could turn off the lights and illuminate the part of the body that I wanted to focus on.

Professional photographers have used similar tricks for years. If you study advertisements and other single-subject photos, you may notice that the point of interest is lighter and more defined than the rest of the photo. Photo filters help alter lighting and color to evoke emotions and thereby influence our arousal levels.

Retail stores and restaurants frequently use lighting, visual patterns, and colors to influence our emotions. A friend who owned a little pizza shop in a fast food court made the simple change of adding a few extra spotlights over the glass food areas. After doing so, he noticed a twenty-five percent increase in sales within the first month. When the world still hosted big conferences, I noticed increased crowds at the booths that brought their own lighting.

When I consulted with teachers, I commonly advised them to minimize wall clutter. When things are lined up at eye level (as you find at an art gallery or library), the eyes move from side to side in rhythm to view items and thus receive calming input. If student artwork is chaotically placed around the room, the eyes don't visually track as rhythmically and sequentially. Instead, the peripheral vision is increasingly stimulated, and the eyes interpret the visual input as more alerting.

Even clothing choices made by a therapist or caregiver can influence the arousal level of those nearby. Bright, fun colors can be energizing, but bold, distinct patterns can be distracting and overly alerting for some. Colors like reds, oranges, and yellows tend to be alerting while blue, greens, and browns tend to be calming.

When we consider how adverse experiences might influence the development of the visual system, we can see how neglect might function to decrease the nurturing experiences that result in strong eye muscles. We can also see how overstimulation of the visual system can lead to habituation, resulting in a child who doesn't attend to important visual input. We can imagine an environment that required hypervigilance to maintain personal safety. It's difficult to turn that off. I imagine that in the future we will also recognize how increased screen time without adequate supervision can also lead to visual deficits. In my own social circle, even after just one year of online pandemic learning, I'm noticing decreased depth perception as just one of the negative impacts of increased screen time. School children aren't practicing looking from the front of the room to the back. They aren't out on a playground searching near and far for friends and sport tools. Their eyes are focused on a singular plane and therefore not getting the needed practice of looking near and far to strengthen the muscles involved in depth perception.

Screens are devoid of the-three dimensional visual cues needed for social connection, language interpretation, and body language. I can only imagine the follow-up studies and how our current generation of school-age children are creating new neural associations we never even imagined just two short years ago.

As we work with children who have difficulty self-calming or self-alerting, I find it useful to understand how the senses are interpreted. Once I have this understanding, my goal is to help structure the environment for these children to give them sensory advantages independent of their abilities. Simple changes like moving a student closer to a window, minimizing clutter on the walls, changing the paint color, or adding a green plant near their desk can have profound effects. In the next section, we will explore additional environmental modifications that can help the child better receive, interpret, and respond to sensory input.

Practical Strategies and Supports

CHAPTER 9

SENSORY DIET SUGGESTIONS

As sensory difficulties become more widely talked about and products to help are more commercialized, there is an increased awareness of sensory diets and strategies. However, many find the specifics of the how-to of sensory diets mysterious. Not everyone reacts to sensation in the same way and there is a wide range of personalization when it comes to our likes and dislikes. Part of what makes

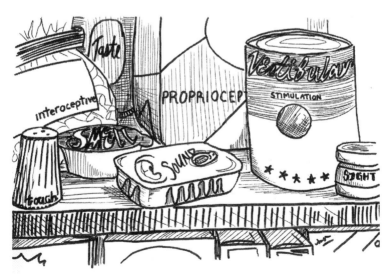

us unique is our sensory preferences. What a boring world it would be if we were all the same.

Sensory processing is constant and multifaceted, and difficult to study. It would be unethical to have studies where the control subjects were denied sensory input. Nothing happens in isolation. Often, multiple sensory systems are engaged simultaneously. It is impossible to restrict sensation, as lack of sensation is itself a sensation. What we have been able to study is general patterns of how people react to types of stimulation and how the brain responds to various types of perceived sensations. As functional brain imaging becomes safer and more widely accessible, we are learning more about sensory interpretation every day.

To understand sensory diets, it is helpful to understand the theory behind the development of these preferences and how both typical and adverse childhood experiences may influence them. As discussed in previous chapters, these preferences start in the mother's womb. The foods the mother eats, the music she listens to, the language she speaks, the movements she makes, all lay the foundation for our sensory development. In very simplistic terms, the body craves what is familiar. Each sensory experience of our development created complex neural pathways that tied together our attachment styles and sensory preferences. But because everyone's experience is different, our preferences will be different. Even biological siblings from the same households will have different preferences. Maybe the oldest child had more one-on-one sensory experiences and possibly a calmer first few years. By the time the third child arrives, there is more chaos, more outside stimulation, and more social connection in their world, starting from their time inside the womb and continuing right through to adulthood. When we consider how early adverse experiences further influence sensory development, these preferences can become even more diverse.

The following recommendations are not meant to be prescriptive, nor are they intended for a child to complete on his or her own. They are meant to be done in the context of a connected relationship. They are a developmental exploration of things that might be helpful to recreate some of the missed neural patterning from early childhood and are designed to help you think through what types of activities will help create more socially functional neural patterns in regard to sensory processing. Like many recipes, sensory diets can be simple or complex. Scrambled eggs are very simple where a souffle requires more skill or consultation with an experienced chef first. For this book, we will focus on the scrambled egg recipes. Most of these recommendations do not require specific training or skill.

FREQUENCY

Repetition facilitates the rewiring of the brain that leads to functional change. The number of repetitions varies per individual and type of task. Sensory rebuilding most often happens in the context of a relationship. Dr. Perry's work has studied how activities that are heavy in repetition, relationship, relevance, reward, rhythm, and respect (The Six Rs) will also increase the effectiveness of the neural response.

When we consider frequency, we look at how long each stimulation lasts before we need another "dose." In her sensory course, Julia Harper, OTR, noted that tactile stimulation lasts two hours, proprioceptive information lasts four hours, and vestibular information lasts six hours. Therefore, throughout the day, the activities should vary a bit. The tactile system will need more repeated doses than the vestibular system. In his book, *What Happened to You?*, Dr. Perry discusses the need for small, frequent, child-controlled doses throughout the day. Several small sensory experiences paired with relationship are better than one structured session once a week. Ideally, there are a few sessions with a skilled provider who can teach you how to make better eggs. Then, you practice your egg skills frequently and playfully between therapy sessions.

We also consider the capacity of the caregiver. Most parents seeking therapeutic services already feel exhausted and defeated, therefore we need to be careful not to further overwhelm them with time-consuming exercises. The activities need to be purposeful, so parents feel they are working toward progress. We need to identify which exercises will target the sensory systems in a developmental sequence based upon the sensory preference/behavior checklists. As OTs focused on functional activity, we then need to identify ways for the family to engage in these sensory-rich experiences within the context of their existing daily activities and routines.

I have found that the best way to set up a successful

sensory diet is to view the child's day through the sensory lens. How can I add vestibular input every six hours with what they are already doing? Having a checklist of prescriptive exercises that the caregiver does through connection and focus every two hours is incredibly valuable. However, it is less valuable if either the caregiver or the child's body language sends a message of frustration and imposition.

In my experience, most caregivers are too overwhelmed to do prescriptive activities every two hours. Therefore, when I recommend a sensory diet, I try and do so more in the context of "tell me your routine and let's find ways to incorporate more mindful sensory experiences and moments of sensory connections together." Instead of spending twenty minutes opening jars of scents, can we take five minutes four times throughout the day to notice the smells around us? What does your shampoo smell like? Is breakfast spicy or bland? What happens when we drink peppermint tea or a cayenne infused juice? Do my bed sheets feel soft or stiff? Do I like to pet my dog behind the ears or on his paws? How is his fur different on different parts of his body? How does my body feel when I jump to get the mail versus spinning? What if I walk while crossing my legs over one another? My goal as the occupational therapist is to teach caregivers things I have noticed clinically in regard to how various activities tend to alert or calm the body. I want parents to understand ways their routines calm or alert their child. I want to work with them to find substitutions and adaptations when needed.

Most people think of needing sensory treatment activities

to calm a person. As we learn more about trauma, we find that many people are dissociating to block out stimuli. For them, we actually need to increase their alertness level while recognizing that their physical state is in hyperarousal. Increasing alerting stimuli for someone who has shut down physically because they are overstimulated is not helpful. It is best to meet these people with a blend of calm and alert. For example, a high BPM song that is played on a low volume. We want to match their hyperarousal rhythm while pairing with calming sensations.

We need to continue to protect our bodies and feel the great sensations of elation and joy. So, my goal is never to provide an entirely calming environment. However, for many children, it is difficult to move smoothly between what we call the arousal continuum, or the states between calm and alert. The goal of the sensory diet is to build new learned experiences of feeling calm and alert while maintaining a sense of connection to both our bodies and other people within each state.

TYPES OF ACTIVITY

When we look at sensory development, we recognize that deep touch is the calming influence over discomfort. Therefore, most sensory diet activities should be paired with sensory input involving deep touch. This may include bending our joints to the midline of the body (clapping our hands together, touching our toes, or hugging our knees), jumping, bumping, crashing, and other deep muscle and skin input stimulation. What proprioceptive or deep touch activities pair well with the task we are attempting? Many sensory courses say that the child will seek the input they need, and I have found this to be true. My job is to allow the child to freely explore the therapeutic space and then encourage connection and sensory pairings that help meet my goals. If my goal is to calm a child and they run in on high alert to the platform swing, I meet them at the swing. I raise the pitch of my voice a bit and maybe wave my arms or bounce my knees to match their tempo. Then, I provide rhythm and connection through bouncing a big therapy ball next to them. Next, I playfully begin to toss the big ball (or maybe a weighted item) towards them to add some rhythmic proprioception. I might start the swing in a tight spin and then gradually pretend we are in a spaceship and begin to make the spin bigger before moving side to side and front to back as we avoid the meteors. Maybe bean bags become meteors that are tossed playfully at the child as more deep touch input. I'm constantly monitoring the child for cues that they don't feel safe and adjusting as needed. Maybe they are the ones throwing the meteors at me or at a target.

A similar activity could happen at home. Maybe the bed is the rocket ship and the pillows are the meteors. Maybe the stuffed animals are on a ship being taken over by pirates and they need to jump to shore. If tolerated, maybe my body behind a pillow becomes a giant crashing wave that bounces into the ship's captain (the child). Once the child is bounced to their belly, I could ask them what sea creature I have become, and we can wiggle our way across the pretend shore sheets (in a connected moment of switching to a more calm movement).

Some parents report to me that when they engage in this type of play, the child can become aggressive or "out of control." After some questioning, I often find that there isn't enough deep touch and proprioceptive input incorporated. The other commonality is that the child is seeking more control and not wanting the adult input to the game. So, I make it more obvious that the child is in control. I give them more simple choices. "Am I a squid or a fish?" "Do you want me to be a meteor or a satellite?" "What color fish am I? What color fish are you?" Sometimes I even try to mimic the playfulness Dr. Purvis brought to the TBRI model with her non-threatening question of, "Whoa, Cowboy! Are you asking? Or are you telling?" I find that as long as I keep my tone friendly and my body language engaged as if they are the leader, my sessions rarely get out of hand.

Another helpful correlation that I have identified is to assess the rhythm of the child-initiated activity. If the child comes in with a very rhythmic movement pattern, that child is trying to calm down. This means that even if they are rhythmically rocking back and forth to a 120 BPM tempo, the child's body is looking to calm down. I'll match that rhythm and help lead them slowly back to calm through co-regulation. When a child is arrhythmic, they are looking to alert. Even if the movements are slow, if they are really sporadic, this indicates to me that the child is tired, bored, or uninterested and is looking for stimulation. I once again match their rhythm and help slowly bring them back up. Maybe I start with a swaggery elephant walk and move towards jumping jacks or jumping through imaginary mud puddles. On occasion, I have a child come in with very high, arrhythmic energy. This child is also seeking stimulation. Intense vestibular input can mimic Ritalin and caffeine as effective ways to help someone focus.

I caution that I am not a physician, and I won't make recommendations about specific medications. I will only say that I have noticed that some children require intense alerting activities in order to move to calm. It is as if they are needing to alert themselves to a level where they finally "feel" alert in order to come back to calm. I find highly vestibular activities paired with intense (but safe) proprioception to be very helpful for these children. The key component is the rhythm. I start out arrhythmic until they find that peak they are seeking and then I switch to a fast relational rhythm that gradually comes back down. When this does not get the result I'm looking for, I might call a physician and see if they could prescribe a short-term medication so that the child gets a chance to pharmaceutically calm to begin to make new associations regarding how calm feels.

I try to keep sensory activities purposeful and appropriately timed. If a child gets anxious before math class, have them do some jumping jacks or wall push-ups before. Could the teacher do these as a class to build community? Could the parent do them as they face the child and mirror the movement? If bath time is too alerting, I look for ways to alter the surrounding sensations. Can we put a heater in the room safely? Can we put towels in the dryer so they are warm when the child gets out? Can we use a calming scented soap? Can we wash the hair by moving the child's chin forward instead of backward? What happens when we add music? So much of a proper sensory diet is simply asking guided questions to help an individual discover things that help them through a daily activity. The following list is a guide to help you ask better questions as you identify ways to help build better neural patterns for socially appropriate sensory functioning.

While it is recommended that caregivers seek an occupational therapist to help them re-train sensory systems, it is helpful to understand the basis behind it. In my experience, the key to successful sensory rehabilitation is understanding how these senses formed in the sequence of human development. As an occupational therapist, I then work safely, with guided activity, to recreate these experiences where the person feels safe and respected. Occupational therapists look at both the person and the environment. The person-centered part involves creating new neural pathways to "re-train" the responses to sensory stimuli. The environment-centered part involves modifying sensory aspects of the child's surroundings to help increase their participation and decrease their anxiety. As caregivers, we don't need fancy degrees or education to provide a fidget toy, weighted blanket, frozen food, scented oils, or different types of chairs. These are scrambled egg recipes. We simply need to have the well-being of the child in mind as we work within relationships to find simple ways to respect their sensory feelings as well as our own. My experience is that as long as the child feels a sense of control, there is little risk

CALMING VERSUS ALERTING ACTIVITIES

VESTIBULAR		PROPRIOCEPTIVE	
Calming	Alerting	Calming	Alerting
Slow position changes	Fast position changes	Flexion (Midline)	Extension (jumping jack "star")
Rhythmic	Arrhythmic	Pushing, pulling, heavy work	Hopping, jumping (trampoline) running
Front to back and side to side swinging	Erratic spinning	Rubbing (deep pressure)	Tickling (Light touch)
Slow movement	Fast movement	Bear hugs	Light kisses
Linear rocking	Spinning	Predictable touch	Unexpected or sporadic touch
Vibration (large amplitude, low frequency - i.e. a ride in a stroller)	Erratic Vibration (i.e a percussion massage)		
Controlled Upside Down Position	Unpredictable Upside Down position		
Push - Pull	Jumping, hitting a pillow		

VISUAL		OLFACTORY	
Calming	**Alerting**	**Calming**	**Alerting**
Balanced/symmetrical decorations on walls	Sporadic, clutter style decorations on walls	Vanilla, cinnamon, lavender	Peppermint, rose, lemon
-	-	-	-
Curves	Jagged points	Sweet	Vile (onion, garlic, cayenne)
-	-	-	
Pastels	Bright colors	Mild foods	-
-	-	-	Spicy foods
Low lighting	Bright lights	Mild odors (baby powder)	-
-	-	-	Strong perfumes, smoke
Light bulbs (new bulbs may flicker less), natural light from windows	Fluorescent lights	Family/familiar	-
	-		Strangers/unfamiliar
	Excessive background		

GUSTATORY	
Calming	**Alerting**

VISUAL		GUSTATORY	
Symmetrical background	Clutter, disorganization	Sweet (increases drooling)	Sour (facilitates lip closure)
-	-	-	-
Linear placements	Strobe effect	Sucking/blowing (midline)	Vertical jaw movement
-	-	-	-
Constant soft light	Disco ball	Milk (allergy caution)	Cold, icy water/ caffeine
-	-	-	-
Round bubble lights and linear string lights	Popping bubbles	Bland	Spicy
-	-	-	-
Blowing bubbles (eyes go to midline)	Movement in the peripheral visual field	Chewy	Crunchy
-		-	-
		Turkey (tryptophan)	Mint, apples

TACTILE	
Calming	**Alerting**
Soft	Prickly
-	-
Deep touch	Light touch
-	-
Neutral warmth	Extreme
-	temperatures
Hard/Smooth	(especially cold)
-	-
Even/congruent	Gooey/Rough
consistency	-
-	Varied consistency
Fake fur	(textured paint)
-	-
Cotton	Sand paper
-	-
Cloth upholstery	Polyester/wool
-	-
Plastic fasteners	Vinyl /leather
-	upholstery
Soft strings/tassels	-
-	Metal/Velcro
Squishy fidgets	fasteners

AUDITORY	
Calming	**Alerting**
Soft, sing-song voice	Erratic yelling
-	-
Rhythmic, quiet	Sudden, arrhythmic,
-	loud
Mind music	-
-	Bass music
Constant pitch	-
-	Pitch changes
Tempo below the	-
heartbeat (40-60	Tempo above the
BPM)	heartbeat (90-120
-	BPM)
Hereditary/familiar	-
music	Unfamiliar or
-	unpredictable music
Soft, melodic music	-
	Loud, irregular
	tempo

BEDTIME	
Calming	**Alerting**
Warm baths (beware	Cold/"prickly"
of bubbles that	showers
"tickle")	-
-	Wool blankets
Sleeping bags	-
-	Stiff new sheets
Heavy, soft blankets	-
-	Sheets tucked
Lots of stuffed	-
animals	A noisy hallway
-	-
Soft or Nature music	Towels without
-	fabric softener
Warm towels in the	
dryer after bath	

GENERAL	
Calming	**Alerting**
Predictable	Non-predictable
-	-
Routine	Change
-	-
Love	Anxiety/fear
-	-
Pleasurable activity	Stressful activity

of harm. For example, a weighted stuffed animal or blanket can be easily added to a bedtime routine. But if the blanket is too heavy for the child to easily remove independently, then it is not a good idea. The sample activities below were created as a list of ingredients that might help create the perfect recipe for a sensory diet. The purpose is to identify which activities a person is engaging in as it relates to their alert or calm tendencies.

SPACE SETUP

Sensory spaces can be simple or extravagant, small or expansive. They can take up an entire gym or be tucked into the corner of a classroom. A simple idea for a small space is to simply attach hooks five feet from the corner of a room and hang twin sheet corners to those hooks. This creates an inexpensive and removable private corner space to calm down. When wanting to contain a mess, a baby pool fits easily inside a zip-up play tent so that plastic balls, rice, and other sensory mediums can be fully explored while keeping the materials contained easily.

One of my favorite sensory spaces for my own home was a "Lycra cloud" in my entry hallway. A few eye bolts screwed into the studs provided a great way to clip up the Lycra sheets. Adding an Amazon wrestling mat on the tile made for a nice little Lycra cloud. I was especially proud of how I hid the eyebolts behind a canvas photo display. There are many self-supporting hammock stands that do not require drilling into walls. Some playground equipment

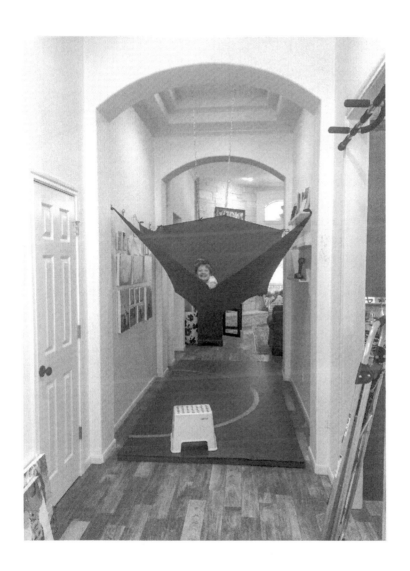

does not involve changing the structure of the room.

Once space and budget are identified, consider layout. The goal of most sensory rooms is to provide access to both alerting and calming input. When working with an overly alert child, the caregiver should first meet them at their energy level, then work to calm within the relationship. The same is true for moving from calm to alert. Keeping alerting spaces more open, and calming spaces more cozy and confined, can maximize the use of the space and provide a way to work through this arousal continuum.

It is beneficial to have stimulation for a variety of senses (tactile, visual, auditory, olfactory, proprioceptive, vestibular). It is best to maintain a calm, streamlined environment that allows more alerting tools to be added as needed. For example, having hooks overhead makes it easy to hang a swing as needed but which can later be stored out of sight. I've seen several OT clinics smartly use the ladder portion of a jungle gym to hang swings. Blues, earth tones, and nature-based images help create a sense of calm. Colorful scarves, ribbons, and bright-colored Lycra can add an alerting element when those tools are used.

When using the space, it's helpful to remember that senses are not stimulated in isolation. For an overly alert client, the caregiver might meet that arousal level through some upbeat music while simultaneously jumping into a ball pit or hopping on a large ball. The alerting music and bright colors of the ball will help the child feel seen while the deep touch and proprioceptive input of the bass in the music and jumping will work to calm the child within the context of the connected relationship. As we look at specific tools and activities within the room, it will be helpful to refer back to the calming versus alerting activity list on page 191.

One of my proud professional accomplishments was co-designing the Simple Sparrow Sequential Relational path with two friends, Jamie Tanner and Trudy Landis. Trudy is the director of Families are Forever and works with All God's Children International. She wanted to create a sensory path that followed the principles of the NMT and TBRI for her friends in Colombia. We had seen sensory paths on the internet and my gut reaction was that some of them looked great. I loved all the movement in the school hallways and the bright, fun graphics and colors. However, many of these paths seemed very alerting to me. There was a disproportionate emphasis on spinning and jumping erratically. We wanted our path to incorporate that sequential progression between calm and alert and to include the crucial element of connection and relationship.

We created a path that highlights side-by-side and mirrored movements that lead users through a sequence of activities that go from alert to calm. The path can also be done in reverse, for individuals that need to progress from calm to alert. Our preliminary feedback has been phenomenal. We have had orders from around the world, and Jamie has now figured out how to print the designs on outdoor, indoor, temporary, and permanent materials. I don't write this to push our product. I mention it to encourage you to be mindful of your own layout and design of the items you choose for your sensory space. Does the flow of the space

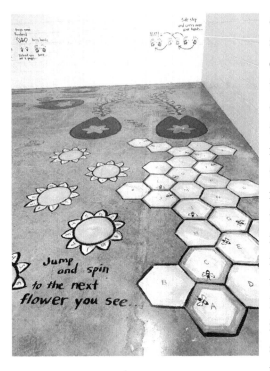

allow for gradual shifts between calm and alert? Are there mirroring opportunities to facilitate co-regulation? Is the design of the room pleasing to look at and inviting for the individuals that will be using it? Is it easy to clean in regard to both sanitation and visual organizing? These are all things we considered as we developed our own progressive pathway to use within our own sensory rooms.

My friend Michael works with horses. He regularly sends me paths that he has created with chalk and items he has in the barn. One of his clients arrives very alert to his session and there is a risk of him running into a busy road as he gets out of the car. Michael uses a sequential path that encourages the child to jump on a horse stick toy along a squiggly line (matching his overly alert state). Then he has to jump from rock to rock and cross his feet rhythmically along a path to begin to bring him to a more neutral state. Towards the end of this path, the child practices deep belly breaths with an expandable ball toy while mirroring Michael in relationship before they begin their session with his horse. Paths don't need to be expensive or fancy. They simply need to be relationally rooted and sensory sequential.

SAFETY

Safety is a big concern with sensory rooms. The caregiver must always provide close supervision and should understand how the equipment is designed to alert or calm. In areas with limited space, a tent can provide the structure of a quiet space but may make supervision difficult. A hole can be cut through the top of the tent for easy supervision. Most children need a sense of control to feel calm. So, the child must have input into the activities. Since children do best with perceived control, a prescriptive checklist is often not helpful. Instead, caregivers can take note of what calms or alerts the child, and offer choices based on those activities. Noticing these preferences and offering a choice of two beneficial activities can help children feel empowered as a part of their sensory plan.

When considering materials, it is important that items are fire-resistant, choke-proof, and non-toxic. Equipment should be securely attached, weight limits considered, appropriate padding or protection provided. Spinning or flashing lights can trigger seizures, so always use caution when spinning a child with a history of seizures. Even a brightly lit window or lamp in the room could cause a strobe type effect for these children when engaged in vestibular spinning activities.

Rolling a ball over a child's belly from head to toe can over-stimulate the vagus nerve and should be avoided. Most other movements where the person is comfortable are harmless for most individuals. Helmets can be added as a level of protection and soft mats on the floor offer added sound dampening and impact-protection. A simple rule that can be helpful is for everyone to "stop" when someone says that word. In my own clinic, this is the only rule. If I tell a child to stop, they must immediately freeze and cease whatever they are doing, because I sense they are in danger. In return, they may tell me to stop (through words or sign language) at any point they feel unsafe due to fear, overstimulation, or simply a lack of desire to engage in the activity. When a child says stop, I make every effort to cease the activity immediately.

WHERE TO BEGIN

A common question is "How do we utilize this room?" It is entirely counterproductive to take an overly alert child and set them loose to spin on a swing in a padded room, then expect them to be independently focused after five minutes. While a sensory room is best utilized with the child's input (children will most often seek what they need), it is important to understand how the continuum from alert to calm progresses.

Considering how the vestibular system influences arousal, I often consider the child through a vestibular lens. Do they show up to my office bouncing off the walls? That child is trying to alert themselves. Are they rhythmically jumping up and down? That child is looking for calm. If it is rhythmic, their body is on a calming trajectory. If it is arrhythmic, it is on the alerting trajectory. For this reason, it works well for the child to choose the first activity upon entering the room.

Based on the child's choice, the caregiver can get an idea of where the child is on that alert-to-calm continuum. The caregiver can then assess if they want the child to be more calm or more alert upon exit, based on the desired social situation. For instance, if a child is lethargic and needs to move next to gym class or a sporting event, the goal would be to help alert them. In this case, the caregiver could guide the child from the calm bubble area to the zipline or trampoline. The caregiver could also change the lighting or music in the room, either of which adjusts the child's environment without the child having to do anything specific. A beneficial practice is an exit routine that is heavy on rhythmic proprioceptive input. It could be something like simply moving a pile of weighted blankets from one bin to the other before the lights are turned out upon exit. Another suggestion is a line of switches that provide a rhythmic and proprioceptive click as the child exits the room.

Before using the room, it would benefit the child and the adult guides to understand which of the activities are alerting and which ones are calm. (Refer to the chart on page 191.) When everyone is in a good calm/alert balance, demonstrate the safe ways that the tools can be utilized and where to find them. Demonstrate how "stop" works and other rules, if necessary, to keep everyone safe.

You can find more tips and resources on my website, http://creativetherapies.com.

Additional Things to Consider When Creating a Sensory Space

- First and foremost, relationships and safety are vital considerations. When possible, provide two of each tool so that the caregiver can mirror the sensory experience. Remember to pair relationally rich deep touch and proprioceptive input alongside alerting input when you are "matching the energy" so that the child doesn't become overly alert.
- A simple soft ball that can be rhythmically passed back and forth or bubbles that can be popped together are easy and natural ways to connect for all ages. These tools also tend to be inexpensive and safe.
- Clear structural boundaries are best. If the room is large, it could be beneficial to incorporate colorful rugs or different wall colors to help visually define the various areas of the room.
- If possible, a door that can close is beneficial to allow for privacy and noise barrier.
- Added textiles such as pillows, canvas prints, and tapestries can also help with noise absorption.
- A space big enough for adult supervision while

allowing the child to freely explore the environment is helpful.

- Provide soft textures when possible. If a hard rocking chair is utilized, provide a washable pillow insert.
- Choose items that are durable and safe. Remember that items might be thrown and that cords may become a choking hazard. Batteries can be swallowed if not securely fastened.
- Weighted blankets or Lycra "silly sacks" can be used independently for self-calming. Be sure that any weighted item is light enough for the child to remove independently.
- Rocking chairs that rock front to back or structures that bounce up and down (i.e., a ball chair or bounce horse) tend to be calming.
- If a child is very alert/agitated, they may need the caregiver to match that energy before they are able to self- or co-calm. An easy way to do this is to play upbeat music while spinning in circles on an office chair. Allow this movement for a few minutes and then encourage more front to back movement as the tempo of the music slows simultaneously.
- Rocking chairs should be heavy enough that a child cannot throw them. Be sure they don't have parts that might pinch little fingers.
- A good sound system with Bluetooth capacity is beneficial for apps such as *Tempo Magic*, which can increase or decrease the level of alerting auditory

stimuli.

- Oil diffusers can be utilized for calming scents such as vanilla, cinnamon, or lavender. For clients that need alerting, peppermint and citrus can wake them up a bit.
- A light projector showing patterns like waves or stars can bring the client's eyes to a focal point and help calm them. Disco balls and laser light shows can be alerting.
- Bongo drums can be used to match a rhythm or tempo with the client as they lead to offer a sense of connection and relationship.
- Soft stuffed animals or even a therapy pet such as a dog or rabbit can offer a living being to provide rhythmic, repetitive soft touch. Animals (even toy stuffed animals) can help children experience relational practice, especially if the child was hurt by a trusted adult.
- Avoid fluorescent lights. If you have no choice, consider adding covers to change the intensity and decrease the flickering effect of the fluorescent bulbs.
- Choose colors that are earth tones or blues to encourage a quiet, alert state. Splashes of color can be added with pillows and other accessories.

Introduction to KALMAR

While teaching in Norway, my friend and colleague, Kaja Johanessen, asked if there was a way to cross-reference patterns in a sensory checklist. Was it possible to create an algorithm that looked at all the sensory preferences and somehow indicated which therapeutic activities would be most likely to create therapeutic change? I began to wonder...

Kaja was brilliant with systems management, relationships, and cognitive goals. But she had difficulty moving a child from the brainstem state of functioning (fight/flight/freeze) to more cortical reasoning. She had excellent strategies and ability to help a child cognitively. But she didn't understand the dosing, the types, the precautions, and which activities would be best to help a child move out of the more brainstem physical functioning. She wanted to figure out how to do somatosensory activities. I later came to realize that many clinicians, even fellow OTs, struggle with these same concepts.

In regard to somatosensory activities, a lot of it is intuitive. It is born out of a confident curiosity of attempting things that "can't hurt and might help" but something I was a natural at. It was something few people have been able to teach. But, with Kaja's encouragement, I was empowered to break down the "whys" behind my OT recommendations. I started looking at the sensory system through a different lens. I started analyzing what my intuition told me to try. This was the birth of the KALMAR tool, an acronym based on the names of the people who helped me develop it: **Kaja,** **A**ne, **L**inn-Marie, **M**arti, **A**nn-Karin, and **R**ob. Together, we launched an online tool that looked at behavioral indications and what activities would most likely encourage brain rehabilitation.

At first, I simply had a giant wall of Post-It notes all over my bedroom wall with sensory behavior symptoms matched with the common OT recommendations. Then, I started to cross reference them so that I could see patterns of common suggested activities that would give a therapist the biggest therapeutic "bang for the buck," so to speak. I felt like I was on a detective TV show like *House, Sherlock,* or *Elementary.* I had connecting strings everywhere. It was a bit of a hot mess. One day, my husband asked why I wasn't simply using the Neurosequential Model Metric as a framework? After all, as the software developer for the app, he had an inside understanding of the algorithms that made it run. Huh…well…that surely does seem like an easier approach. Especially since it is already based off of Dr. Perry's brilliance and understanding of the brain's sequential functionality.

So, we sought the blessing and approval to borrow some of the principles of the metric. I am not a psychologist, and the frontal cortex is not my specialty. Nor do I believe I'm capable of developing remediation techniques for cognitive based interventions. But I do know the sensory system and areas of the brain that pertain to somatosensory function. It was a perfect base for me to pick and choose some of the same domains that I was comfortable with and start developing activity recommendations.

Occupational therapists specialize in activities. I LOVE a good activity analysis. Funny story, I really disliked activity analysis exercises in OT school. I remember almost walking out of the degree program my first year when the instructor asked us to write a minimum fifty-step process for making toast. What the heck? You put the bread in, push the button, make toast. Why would I possibly want to make more work for myself by making these three steps so much more complicated?

Well, as I learned from my ever-patient instructor, when we know how much goes into an activity, we can better diagnose where the glitch/dysfunction lies so that we can rehab the person. If a person can't use two hands to remove the bread from the wrapper, they will never get to the part of putting it into the toaster. If they can't rotate their wrist to turn the dial to the desired cooking level, they will not enjoy their toast. If they can't remember to take the toast out, they will have cold toast and the butter will not spread. If they can't reach over their head due to a shoulder injury, they may not be able to get the bread high enough to place in the toaster slot.

I finally understood that nothing is as simple as it seems. Every "activity of daily living" (ADL) has many components. When we are able to successfully analyze these components, only then will we be able to know how to target our healing, remediation, or rehab. The sensory system is simply really complicated toast. I'm grateful for my degree in occupational therapy that has prepared me to start breaking it into the thousands of steps it involves to better help caregivers help kids whose sensory systems have a step that they need help with. When we add a layer of complex trauma, adverse developmental experiences, and protective developmental tendencies, it becomes even more steps to analyze. That slice of toast becomes Texas toast.

I began to break down the steps and things that influenced the skills being assessed in common areas of concern such as sleep, nutrition, attachment, fine motor skills, coordination, and mood. I created a rating scale for which therapeutic activities would target rehabilitation of those concerns. If you go to this website, http://kalmar.creativetherapies. com/, you will find a list of questions that are related to sequential brain development from an OT perspective, the things OTs typically address in a treatment session. As you answer the severity of the concern, or Koncern, Rob's code cross references activities that would be helpful and figures out which ones will give you the biggest bang for your buck. It calculates the activity selection through my understanding of Dr. Perry's neurosequential model of brain hierarchy, state dependent function, and development. The activity suggestions are rooted in TBRI principles of connecting and empowering. It is my attempt at giving parents, educators, counselors, and other therapists ideas to begin helping children who have experienced adversity heal.

When developing this tool, we decided to not save results or require identifying information. Our reasoning for this was to keep the cost down. If we saved information, we would have to add extra securities for privacy and medical compliance regulations. We didn't want to have to pass that cost along to our users. We wanted to keep it an accessible, easy to use, free resource. The user guide is on the home page. Most people find it very simple and you can change your answers and re-submit as many times as is helpful. One simple suggestion I have is to try and give the child the benefit of the doubt. The fewer number of "Koncerns" you have, the more targeted the activity suggestions will be for that specific concern. For some clients, I recommend filling it out a few times. The first time, target only the most severe concerns. The next time, do a more general overview and see if the order of suggestions changes drastically. In general, as the website explains, the more systems that are involved, the more brainstem-focused the activities will be. Since it was based off the NMT model, it is important to build the foundations before we start working on higher level activities. We hope you find it helpful.

SIMPLE SPARROW BACKSTORY

I have some pretty amazing friends. Like me, they are trying to make the world a little bit better for others. Like me, they have their own trauma backgrounds, and have found healing that they want to share with others. Jamie Tanner is one of those friends. When we first met, we both were very busy and weren't looking to get closer to anyone. We were young moms simply trying to get through the long days and working through our own backgrounds. Our "friend cards" were already fully punched.

Jamie had discovered that being on a farm was healing for her. So, she convinced her husband to move from the city to a two-acre plot of land just north of Austin. Our social circles overlapped often, but we didn't connect until spring of 2015. That's when my daughter had LOTS of questions about where babies come from.

Loving anatomy and being very scientifically blunt, I was happy to make very simplistic models out of playdough and very simplified drawings for my daughter. I thought I was handling the questions beautifully. My child, however, wanted DETAILS. Like really personal and specific details. One of the questions was, "Do people ever watch when babies are made?" Ummmmm….. Ahhhhhh…. I promised to always answer honestly. But I was **confident** she didn't want the dark truth to that question. I was proud of my quick response of, "Well, that's not really a great idea. It's really meant to be personal and special between people who love each other." To which she replied, "Can I watch you and Daddy?" Uh, "That's a hard 'No.'" More quick thinking and I remembered my acquaintance, Farmer Jamie. I called her up and asked if she had any bunnies that she wanted to breed. She did. Phew! That was resolved pleasantly.

My daughter spent all of five seconds peeping at the bunnies and her curiosity was satisfied. Until the next day when she asked how the babies would be making their exit. As luck would have it, Jamie had a goat about to give birth. She graciously opened her barnyard up for us to witness the miracle of birth. Being new to goat births, Jamie was convinced the birth due date would be a small window. She was an army nurse medic and had experienced four natural births of her own. So, when this goat was very overdue and had birth complications, we were caught by surprise. It was a pretty traumatic event. Children were escorted to the house to protect their little hearts. Thankfully, my daughter Suzy had seen enough of the process that her curiosity was satisfied.

While we waited on this goat, we bonded. We experienced something new and difficult *together*. We got through it *together*. I was her buddy. This traumatic experience brought us closer together. Because we had each other, our resilience grew within the context of relationship. I made new neural pathways that day for understanding that I can do hard goat birth things. And I made a new best friend in the process. If you want more of the comical details, we have a podcast about the "Birth of Simple Sparrow" on my Podbean channel, martiot.podbean.com.

Several weeks after our goat birth foundation, I was caring for some baby bunnies born on the farm. You can guess which ones. These would become the bunnies mentioned in Chapter 7 who helped my client who had trouble finding her voice.

About this same time, I was struggling with the concepts of being a connected parent and having enough to give my own family. I wanted to practice what I preached. I didn't want to be someone who told her clients to put the phone down and spend time with their child when I was constantly flying all over the world without my own children, who needed attachment repair work.

After some heartfelt conversations with my husband, we agreed I would slow down my work schedule. I would become a theatre costume mom and a baseball dugout mom. Maybe I'd even cook a few meals each week to show my husband some connection, too. Jamie was curious if others would find healing at that farm. She reached out to do classes with at-risk youth at the local high school. She partnered with a home for women who had been trafficked. She transported baby chicks and rabbits to an assisted living facility.

Jamie was seeing firsthand how animals could help people. With the help of a generous friend, we co-founded Simple Sparrow care farm in 2016. I felt a strong sense that I was supposed to put aside my professional career and use my time to move to the background and support others, especially Jamie. She didn't "need" my help. She's a very strong, courageous, and capable woman. My help was simply a bonus for her. My name may have opened a few doors. But the room was hers once she was inside.

As I was stepping down from seminar teaching, I decided to "go out with a bang" at the Neurosequential Symposium in Banff. I bought 100 yards of Lycra and prepared for a massive Lycrapalooza event with my fellow trauma treaters. We had a blast. We met new friends and caught up with old friends.

We were invited on a hike which led to a career-changing conversation with Chelle Taylor, a brilliant and compassionate psychologist in Australia. She asked if I would consider training in Australia. My husband quickly confirmed that I would happily come out of retirement for a speaking engagement in Australia. We could take the whole family. Diving the Great Barrier Reef was a mutual goal for us.

I still felt convinced that I was supposed to be behind the scenes promoting the care farm. In an incredible and inspiring twist of events, I discovered the organization who would be sponsoring me in Australia was planning to launch…a care farm. Except, care farming was a brand new concept to their area and they were eager to understand more about how nature, farming, animals, and the sensory system can bring holistic healing. Wow. That's divine, right there. I just so happened to know someone who was researching care farming for her masters degree. Jamie even had family that lived in Australia. Profound.

Jamie spent the next six months diving deeper into the history (mostly in Europe) of care farming. Jamie poured her heart into program planning and community outreach. We launched the concept of collaborative care farming in Australia in 2019. We made new lifelong friends down under and I fed a kangaroo. Not a bad way to enjoy retirement.

As of this writing, I've stepped down from the Simple Sparrow board simply because we wanted to put limits on board terms to keep the board fresh. I'm still best friends with Jamie and I visit the farm often, especially when there are baby bunnies that need holding. We are in conversations about building a sensory room and providing trainings on the property. It really is a magical place to learn, grow, and heal.

I have seen firsthand and read the research about animal-assisted therapy. I've seen how animals can provide rhythmic, relational, repetitive, respectful, and relevant sensory input. When someone is hurt by a human, an animal can be a safe bridge to a therapeutic relationship. I've seen a child who wasn't cared for learn to care for an animal, and in turn, learn to care for himself and others. I've seen individuals who feel unskilled find the pride of growing something beautiful. I've seen children who feel unworthy accept the unconditional love of a dog. I've seen adolescents who don't trust give respect to a guard llama. I've seen women who haven't been able to consistently show up for a job arrive early to care for animals that they know depend on them.

I've seen Jamie simply provide a cup of tea, an empathetic ear, and a fuzzy bunny or rabbit to hold while a mother processes the grief of losing a child. I've seen how nature can be an adjunct to nurture. I've seen that relationships with animals can lead to relationships with people. On only two acres. Care farming doesn't have to be fancy. It doesn't have to be expensive. It can be as simple as a pet rabbit in the school counselor's office. Jamie recognized this and began an animal loan/adoption program with one of the local schools. One of my favorite stories is of a student who had a poor attendance record. After being introduced to the rabbit and being given responsibility to check the rabbit before school each day, the student hasn't had a single unexcused absence.

Simple Sparrow uses both animals and plants as treatment activities. The pulling of weeds provides rich rhythmic and repetitive proprioceptive information with the visual appeal of progress. Jamie helps people plant seeds and then connects with them when they return for another visit by asking how their plant is growing. Growing something from a tiny seed takes time and provides opportunity for social interaction as we evaluate the progression of growth over time. We can talk about how some plants have thorns to protect themselves but still produce the most beautiful, fragrant flowers. We simply need to be careful how we interact with them. We find safe ways to get close with plants as we explore safe ways for others to get close to us.

Farmyards and other outdoor areas are rich with somatosensory opportunities. When we look at the arousal continuum, we understand how those rhythmic, repetitive, relevant activities help build the neural foundations for self-regulation and working towards a soothing state of calm. As you work to find activities to help children who have experienced adversity, I encourage you to look outside. If you don't have space to work outside, I encourage you to bring nature indoors. Not everyone does great with a jumpy little baby bunny. If a child hasn't mastered "gentle," a tiny chick might not be the best animal to start with. This is one of the reasons Jamie likes her goats. Goats have short hair that doesn't pull easily, and they tend to be pretty pain resistant. Not only is it difficult to pinch and pull their tough skin and fur, they tend to be more amicable to the occasional learning interaction with children who have not yet learned the term "gentle." If the child's eyes are prone to notice peripheral movement and be alerted by that, a dog or chicken will likely not be the best therapy animal. Turtles and snakes tend to move very slowly and encourage a more focal vision. For some children who tend to be on the more alert side of the continuum, chickens can be great for matching that energy initially. Some plants require daily monitoring and soil checks. They can be great motivation for someone to have the motivation to get out of bed and check on the plant. Some plants are easily cared for and don't require as much care. These plants are better for someone who feels shame and might be upset if the plant did not grow well. At Simple Sparrow, we look at the goals of our clients and help to match them with the farming activity that will help them reach that goal within our community. Our clients work the land, connect with the animals, care for the plants, and then proudly share the fruits of their labor with neighbors in our community.

Care farms provide opportunities to tell stories and relate to animals. Some children can find parallels to their own stories as they connect to the farm animals and plants. We have animals who have been adopted. We have animals who have limb differences. We have animals who are excitable and animals that are lower energy. Jamie even talks about seeds and how they can be cast aside by the wind or fall to the ground after riding along in an animal's fur. But that seed can then bloom where it is planted. That seed starts out hard and plain and grows into something beautiful and even nourishing to others.

Stories are how we remember and how we often frame who we are and what we have experienced. For many, trauma is a dark chapter in their life story. They long to change the plot of their historic stories. Telling stories about farm concepts and animals can be a unique way to help children who have experienced adversity learn to view their stories with resilience. Through relationships with the land and animals, we can help these children create new stories of empowerment and connection. To learn more about our simple care farm, visit us in person or online at www.simplesparrow.farm.

Conclusion

I'm so grateful that Dr. Cross encouraged me to write this book. He told me it could help others and I'm so hopeful he is right. Maybe someone will read it and not feel so alone or shameful about their own struggles. I'm grateful for a life well lived and full of interesting stories and experiences. I'm grateful I've had so many buddies to buffer the adverse experiences of my life. I'm grateful for the way I've developed and the insight it has given me in regard to living outside of "normal."

I hope this book has given you some things to think about as you help children who have experienced adversity.

I hope it is part of the current culture change from being trauma-informed to trauma-transformed or trauma-responsive.

I hope you try some things that "can't hurt, might help."

I hope you can repair relationships and experiences that will make your children interesting.

I hope you don't give up on any child that crosses your path. There is always hope for improvement if we simply adjust our expectations instead of giving up.

I hope this book helps you consider that we are all doing the best we can with what we are capable of. We are capable of more when we have relational connections.

ACKNOWLEDGEMENTS

I'm so grateful that I can look back in my life and see ways I was blessed with just the right people at just the right moments. I had many beautiful, loving women in my life who poured into me.

In my teen years, Christine Davis, my first mother-in-law, accepted me into her home and raised me alongside her son.

In my twenties, Deb Dallman practically adopted me. I was a terrible cook and she had three kids in different schools. We traded carpool service for home cooked dinners followed by quilting and family fellowship. I looked at her family and marriage as the model I would strive for. Although I grew up in the church, she taught me who Jesus really was and how to love others so well. She is probably one of the most influential people in my life.

In my thirties, I had Carolyn Bryant. We met at the neighborhood park as our children toddled awkwardly on the playground equipment. She became my greatest confidant and saving grace as I navigated parenting as an expert without any answers.

In my forties, I met Deana Boggess. She taught my children in kindergarten and adopted them as a grandmother's influence. Deana introduced me to the Special Needs Ministry and has taught me about compassion and acceptance through her life example.

A few years ago, a colleague, Annie Chase, OTR, formed a Facebook group for OTs working in the field of trauma. It is here that I discovered a community of therapists who pour into each other as we pour into people with adverse life experiences. I met Holly Timberline, OTR, and Teri Barney, OTR, in this group — two women who have helped me create this book. Holly, especially, has spent countless hours reading and helping me re-word every paragraph. If you found this book easy to read, it is because of Holly. To have someone who excels at both trauma informed OT and editing feels like a gracious divine intervention. The women in the Trauma Informed OT Facebook group have supported and encouraged me. They've been my buddies as we work to change systems and figure out really hard cases. Kaja Johanessen, Michelle Gerbode, Chelle Taylor, Susie Meadows, Heather Hopper, Barb Ford, Krista Soria, Sarah Mercado, Jan Croft, and Julie Kouri have been so influential in my journey as a pediatric therapist.

Special thanks to the following people who are such an important part of my personal life as well as my professional one:

Michael Remole, thank you for being so encouraging to me and my family. To know you is to know acceptance, enthusiasm, and Christ's love. I look forward to your frequent texts, memes, videos, and constant encouragement and example of continually striving to make the world better for others.

Thank you to my parents and siblings for giving me an interesting life and stories worth telling.

Thank you, Bruce, for calling me so many years ago and blessing my family and other families around the world in so many ways through your work. Thank you for giving my sweet Rob a way to use his talents to serve others without having to talk to them. Thank you for creating a community of helpers who have developed deep relationships because of your vision and introduction in the beautiful Canadian Rockies. Your place of connection has truly connected others in impactful ways.

Thank you, Dr. Cross, for giving me the initial nudge to write this book. Without your blessing and encouragement, I would never have had the courage to create this. Thank you for validating me, praising me, and being so gracious as you share your life's work with others around the world.

My Mom Squad and Dinner Darlings have been my behind-the-scenes cheerleaders and counselors. You have given me a place to be authentic and vulnerable and I'm so grateful for your unconditional love, confidence, and support.

Hope, thank you for being so gracious with me as I tested out these new TBRI principles on you as a teenager. Thank you for your forgiveness and patience with the many do-overs as we unpacked some of those shipping boxes together. I love you and am so grateful God brought you back into our lives.

Thank you, especially, to my Smith family. Suzy, you were my inspiration to learn more about the neurobiology of trauma. I hope and pray that our relationship will remain strong, and we will continue to do the work together for the repairs that will come up. I'm so incredibly proud of you. You are enough, just as you are. You were wonderfully made and able to overcome difficult circumstances and situations. I believe in you! Andy, thanks for being my sidekick through this crazy journey of life. I love your sense of humor and big feelings. I hope you always share your amazing hugs with me. Finally, to My Sweet Rob... You are my favorite favorite. Without you, my life would be drastically different and not nearly as fun, or functional. Thank you for believing in me, knowing me, encouraging me, caring for me, funding me, and loving me so well. Thank you for allowing me to truly know and love you in return. Thank you for making me laugh and being the most amazing partner to me and father to our children. We are all so blessed to be with you. Loves you.

ABOUT MARTI

Marti Smith, OTR/L is an occupational therapist who specializes in teaching how sensory activities relate to trauma. She is a fellow with ChildTrauma Academy, a TBRI practitioner, creator of the KALMAR App, and co-founder of Simple Sparrow care farm. She resides in Austin, Texas with her family and enjoys speaking, traveling, hiking, off-roading, photography, quilting, baking cookies, and studying neuroscience. Her friends call her the Lycra Princess and she loves creatively collaborating with colleagues around the world to help children and families who have experienced adversity.

For more about Marti, please visit http://creativetherapies.com.

Made in the USA
Columbia, SC
18 May 2021